Professional Makeup Artistry
Student Workbook

School of Makeup Artistry

Women in Gear, LLC

SUPPLEMENT WORKBOOK FOR ONLINE COURSE

This book intended to be used with the online pro makeup artistry course found at www.womeningear.com.

CONTENTS

Introduction

Getting paid to be a professional makeup artist is a rewarding career that other people will envy. Regardless of the fact that most women wear makeup, a makeup artist is needed for those attending upscale events, brides who need professional wedding makeup. There are so many opportunities to do makeup and the prospects are limitless.

Turning your love of makeup artistry into a career can be a smart decision.

As a professional freelance makeup artist student, you will learn the correct way to apply makeup to other people, you will learn the tricks of the trade to create the perfect look for any occasion and you will have the opportunity to work with many different clients and in many different environments. You will get to use your makeup skills to achieve the look each client is searching for and you will have the skill to apply the dramatic look a photographer is trying to capture. Your new found talents will mean you can enhance the essence of each person you get the pleasure of working with and it will be your job to accomplish what others are unable to achieve. Being a professional makeup artist will allow you to work with a variety of clients that will need an expert to do their makeup. The face is your canvas and makeup is your medium.

This manual will serve as a guide as you progress through your makeup artistry course. No matter where your makeup artist skills take you when you complete your makeup artistry course this manual will be a handy reference. Maybe you're interested in owning your own business or want to work in an upscale salon, you might even want to work within the growing global beauty spectrum for a large cosmetics company? If so this manual and your makeup artistry course can help you get a start on your new career path.

It's time to embark on an exciting career in the world of makeup artistry.,

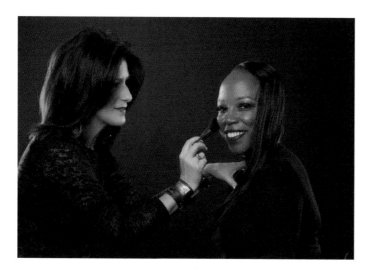

History of Makeup

Throughout history many civilizations used numerous forms of cosmetics, though not always recognizable as cosmetics used today, they were in fact viewed as an enhancement. For centuries these cosmetic enhancements were used in religious rituals to enhance the beauty of the person and to promote good health.

Cosmetic usage throughout history was practiced for many reasons and often times to promote civilizations practical concerns, a class system, or simply to enhance a person's beauty. No matter what reason ancient civilizations used cosmetics; their desire to enhance the facial and body features still persist today and has become a multi-billion dollar industry.

COSMETICS IN THE ANCIENT WORLD

10,000 BC
Men and women in Egypt use scented oils and ointments to clean and soften their skin and mask body odor. Cosmetics were an integral part of Egyptian hygiene and health, oils and creams were used for protection against the hot Egyptian sun and dry winds. Myrrh, thyme, marjoram, chamomile, lavender, lily, peppermint, rosemary, cedar, rose, aloe, olive oil, sesame oil, and almond oil provided the basic ingredients for most perfumes that Egyptians used for religious rituals.

4000 BC
Egyptian women applied galena mesdemet (made of copper and lead ore) and malachite (a bright green paste of copper minerals) to their faces for color and definition, as well they employed a combination of burnt almonds, oxidized copper, coppers ores, lead, ash, and ochre combined together to create Kohl to adorn their eyes in the iconic almond shape. Egyptian women often carried cosmetics to parties in makeup boxes and kept them under their chairs much like today's makeup cases.

3000 BC
The Chinese began to stain their fingernails with gum Arabic, gelatin, beeswax, and egg and the colors they used represented a social class: Chou dynasty royals wore gold and silver, with subsequent royals wearing black or red. During this time lower classes were forbidden to wear bright colors on their nails.
During this same period, Grecian women painted their faces with white lead and applied crushed mulberries as rouge. The application of fake eyebrows, often made of oxen hair, is also fashionable.

1500 BC
Chinese and Japanese citizens commonly use rice powder to make their faces white. Eyebrows were shaved off, teeth painted gold or black and henna dyes were applied to stain their hair and faces.

1000 BC
Grecians whiten their complexion with chalk or lead face powder and fashioned crude lipstick out of ochre clays laced with red iron.

EARLY COSMETICS

100 AD
In Rome, people put barley flour and butter on their pimples and sheep fat and blood on their fingernails for polish. In addition, mud baths came into vogue, and some Roman men dye their hair blond.

300-400 AD
Henna was used in India as a hair dye and mehndi, an art form in which complex designs are painted on to the hands and feet, especially before a Hindu wedding, was used to decorate the skin. Henna was also used during this era in some North African cultures.

COSMETICS IN THE MIDDLE AGES

1200 AD
As a result of the Crusades, perfumes arrive in Europe from the Middle East. The beginning of the import trade included cosmetics and perfumes.

1300 AD
In Elizabethan England, dyed red hair comes into fashion. Society women wear egg whites over their faces to create the appearance of a paler complexion. Yet, some thought cosmetics blocked proper circulation and therefore posed a health threat.

RENAISSANCE COSMETICS

1400 - 1500 AD
In Europe, only the aristocracy use cosmetics with Italy and France emerging as the main centers of cosmetics manufacturing. It is also the time when arsenic begins to show up in face powder instead of lead. The modern notion of complex scent making evolves in France and early fragrances are amalgams of naturally occurring ingredients. Later, chemical processes for combining and testing scents supersede their arduous and labor-intensive predecessors. French perfumeries are born.

1500-1600 AD
European women often attempt to lighten their skin using a variety of products including white lead paint. Queen Elizabeth I of England was well known for her use of white lead, with which she created a look known as "the mask of youth." Blonde hair rises in popularity and mixtures of black sulfur, alum, and honey was painted onto the hair and left to work in the sun.

19TH AND 20TH CENTURY COSMETICS

1800 AD

Zinc oxide becomes widely used as a face powder replacing the previously used deadly mixtures of lead and copper. One such mixture called ceruse that is made from white lead, is later discovered to be toxic and blamed for physical problems including facial tremors, muscle paralysis, and even death.

During this era, Queen Victoria publicly declared makeup improper and view it as vulgar and acceptable only for use by actors.

1900 AD

In Edwardian Society, pressure begins to increase in middle-aged women to appear as young as possible while maintaining publicly a no-hassle appearance. This begins a trend of secretly using cosmetics to achieve this goal.

Later 1900 AD

Beauty salons increase in popularity, though patronage of such salons was not necessarily accepted, many women loathe admitting that they needed assistance to look young, so they often entered salons through the back door.

Thus the phrase "slipping through the back door" was born.

2000 AD

Today we are a society thriving on beauty and cosmetics. In 2012 Vanity Fair reported that $17 billion dollars was spent on makeup in the United States and women purchase two times more makeup than they will ever need or use.

Today the average woman owns

7 Lipsticks but use only 2 of them on rotation
12 Eye shadows but only use 5 of them on rotation
2-3 Mascaras but only use 1
3 forms of blush in various shades but only use 1
2 foundations and they use one or both daily

So it appears women own more than need and there's a demand to look and stay beautiful in today's growing social media society. This is good news for aspiring makeup artists.

Brushes-Implements-Tools

Why are makeup brushes, implements, and tools so important to makeup artists?

Makeup brushes come in all shapes and sizes and choosing the right makeup brush is important, each brush has a specific purpose and that purpose creates the finished product. Using a quality brush for the right purpose will make a significant difference during the application process. Brushes are made in three different parts: the handle, the ferrule (the metal part that holds it together) and the bristles. Makeup brush bristles can be synthetic or natural. The most popular blends are the natural blends that consist of sable, squirrel, mink, goat or pony hair. Investing in a good set of brushes will last you years and your finished product will show up as a good investment.

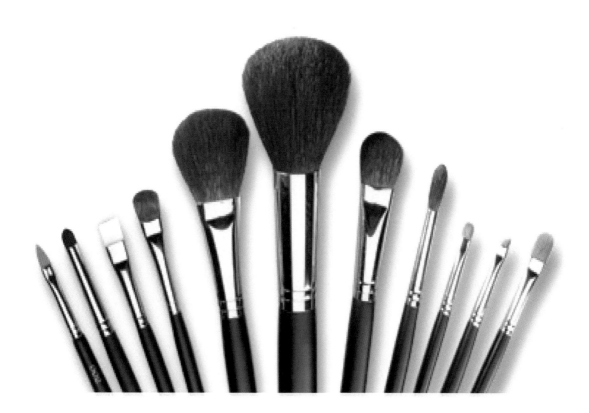

Let's Review Makeup Brushes

Powder Brush: Can come in all shapes, but are always the larger brush out of the bunch. This brush is used for applying powder foundation or blush and it is a great tool for blending products to achieve a flawless finish.

Blush Brush: Typically come rounded or angled they are smaller then powder brushes and are designed to cover the cheek area of all face shapes and sizes.

Concealer Brush: Is a firm flat brush and is used to conceal blemishes as well as around the upper and lower eye area.

Basic Eye Shadow brush: This is a softer flat brush designed to pick up an ample amount of eye shadow to press and pack on the eyelid, at the same time this brush is made to blend shadows to soften and get a desired look.

Crease Brush: This brush is usually made with coarser hair and is smaller and rounder in appearance. It is perfect for that ever-so-sexy smoky eye look.

Eyeliner brush: These brushes are very fine but are made with firm bristles. The firm bristles help achieve the perfect thin pencil look or thick sexy cat eye. It's great for hitting right in and above the lash line creating a full coverage finish.

Brow Brush: This brush has firm thin bristles and is angled. It can be used to fill in a brow or to apply eyeliner.

Lash & Brow Comb: One side has a comb used to remove excess mascara and the other side has a brush to smooth out brows before or after powder application. Some lash/brow combs come with a metal comb side and others are plastic.

Lip Brush: Is very similar to a concealer brush but much smaller and tapered with a rounded edge. It is designed to apply lipstick or lip-gloss.

Implements and Tools

Lash Curler: A lash curler is great for a client who has straight lashes. When used correctly you can achieve a natural curled look.

Pencil Sharpener: Eyeliner pencils and lip pencils are usually made of soft wax-like material and can break easily. With this being said you can easily see why it's important to have a sharpener on hand. Keeping your lip liners and eyeliners sharpened will allow for easy application.

Hair Bands & Clips: Being able to see your client's full face during a makeup application is crucial. It is important to have hair bands and clips readily available to push or pull all hair away from the clients face. Before showing the client her finished look remove all clips and bands to highlight your work.

Makeup Cape or Towel: Protect your client's clothing before starting makeup application to ensure your client gets the makeover not their clothing.

Makeup Brush Tool Belt: Make your life easier with ease of access to your tools and brushes. A professional tool belt made exclusively for your brushes will make your life as a Makeup Artist so much more efficient.

Cleaning Agent: Proper sanitation must be practiced to keep you and your client safe. This cleaning agent will be used to clean your hands, surfaces, and tools. Disinfecting wipes can be used for surfaces and tools and sanitizer for your hands.

Facial Cleanser: It is ideal to have your client show up with a freshly washed and moisturized face. But if they don't show up for their appointment with a clean face, always have a gentle face wash on hand. You can always use the quick face wipes found online or at your drugstore.

Color wheel: To help assist with choosing the right colors for your client's skin tone.

Disposable Tools

Tissues: Tissues are a great tool for blotting powder or lipstick. It can also be used to protect under the eyes when applying shadow so it does not sprinkle on to the skin below.

Q-Tips: Are perfect for fixing mistakes. They are great for removing mascara and any other smudges that may occur during the application process.

Spatulas: Used to remove concealer or scrape lipstick from jars and containers. Never dip your fingers into products or apply them directly to your clients face. Spatulas are essential to help keep all your makeup free of bacteria and your client safe from cross contamination.

Mascara Wand: To prevent cross-contamination use disposable mascara wands when applying mascara. Never double dip your wands in the mascara tube, and use a new wand for each application.

Lip Gloss Wand: To prevent cross-contamination use lip wands when applying lip-gloss. Never double dip your wand in a tube of lip-gloss, use a new wand for each application.

Foundation Sponge Applicator: These triangular disposable foundation sponges are great for one-time use and should be in every makeup artist kit.

Artist Palette: When you have decided on the colors you will be using on your client put the amount you need on to your palette. Since all the products you need will be right there on your palette it will help maximize your time for makeup application and keep you safe from accidental cross-contamination. Palettes can be found online or at your local craft store.

Cleaning Your Makeup Brushes

As a makeup artist, it is your responsibility to keep your makeup brushes and tools cleaned and sanitized. So cleaning your makeup brushes after every use is key to keeping your clients safe from harmful bacteria.

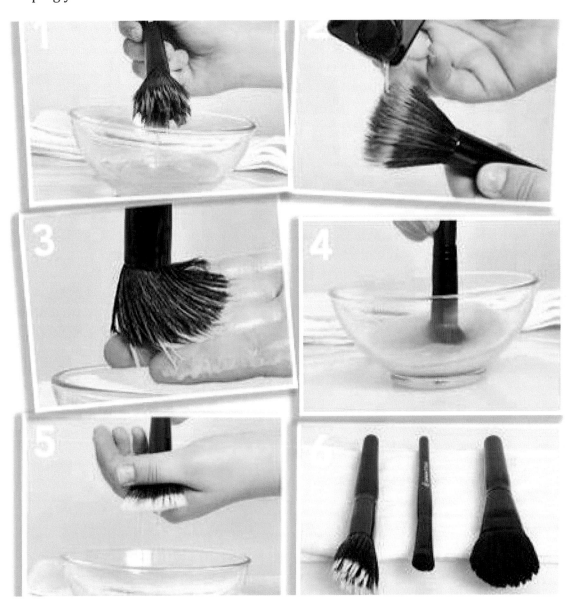

Client Safety & Sanitation

Talking about or even thinking about infection issues is never a fun subject but the importance of this topic for you the Makeup Artist and your clients is crucial to your business and the knowledge gained on this very serious topic can help you be the best in your field.

Disinfection Rule: *If you can't disinfect then dispose of!*

Bacteria: are one-celled organisms that have both plant and animal characteristics Bacteria can live on makeup tools and cause a variety of infections, one we are all most familiar is called a blemish. It is your responsibility as a makeup artist to ensure that your client safe. The makeup artist should have an understanding of potentially harmful organisms to ensure client's safety and having a clear view of infection control will help reduce or eliminate the transmission of organisms that are infectious.

Failure to practice proper storage, safe handling, and complete sanitation of products and implements can cause many serious problems. One such problem is acne as well as other more serious conditions such as infestations that can cause rosacea, boils, or loss of eyelashes or brows, pink eye, staph, and even herpes.

Prevention First

Always take precautions for the safety of you the Makeup Artist and your clients.

Proper hand-washing technique: Wash hands with warm water and antibacterial soap, work the soap into the groves and folds of your hands for twenty seconds and rinse thoroughly then drying hands completely.

Use hand sanitizer throughout your makeup service

- Thoroughly cleanse clients skin before applying makeup
- Do not share applicator tools between clients
- Use a metal palette
- Clean reusable tools with alcohol
- Use professionally formulated brush cleaner to clean brushes

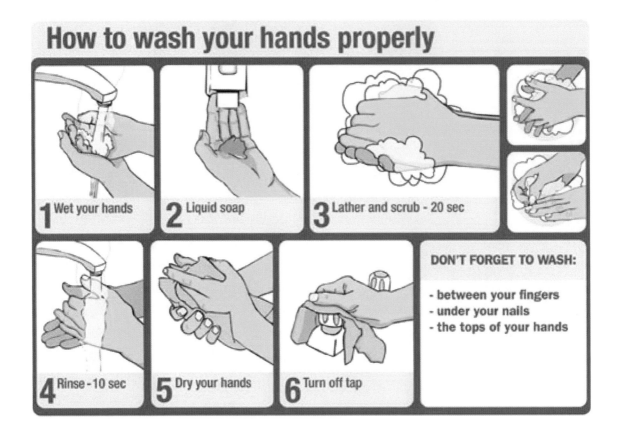

Exposure Incidents

You should never perform Makeup Artistry procedures on a client who has open wounds or abrasions on the skin or any noticeable disease or infection.

Blood Spill Procedure

- Stop the service
- Put on gloves to protect yourself
- Stop the bleeding by applying pressure with clean cotton or gauze.
- When bleeding has stopped, clean injured area with antiseptic.
- Bandage the cut with adhesive bandage.
- Clean and disinfect workstation using an EPA registered disinfectant designed for cleaning blood.
- Discard all contaminated items in a double bag labeled "bio-hazard"
- Before removing your gloves make sure all contaminated tools have been thoroughly cleaned and completely immersed in an EPA registered disinfectant for 10 min or for the time recommended on the label. Be sure you do not touch other work surfaces, such as faucets, counters. If you do that area must be thoroughly cleaned as well
- Remove your gloves and dispose of them in the double bag labeled "bio-hazard"
- Recommend the client see a physician if signs of redness or swelling occur

When in doubt do not perform the Makeup Application Service and never Double Dip

Color Theory

Understanding Color and the Color Wheel

Fact: Understanding color theory will make you a better makeup artist!

Once you have completed this section you will have a thorough understanding of basic color theory and you will know how to use the color wheel effectively for makeup applications on your clients.

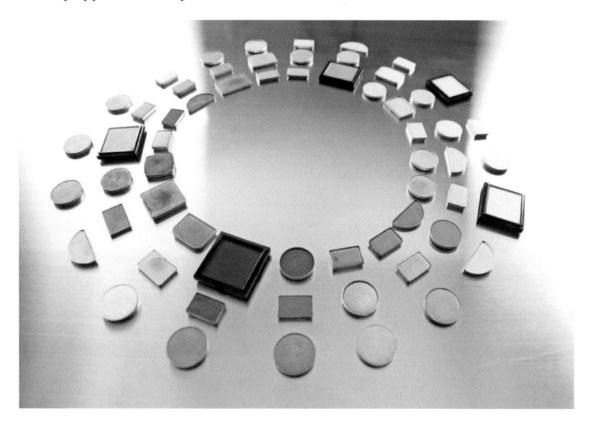

Color Terminology

With colors you can set a mood, attract attention or make a statement. There is a proven psychology behind colors and they can tell stories. By selecting the right color scheme, you can create an ambiance of elegance, warmth or tranquility or you can convey an image of playful youthfulness.

Hue- I when a color is at its maximum intensity.
Tint – Anytime white is added to a pure hue it is referred to as tinting.
Shade- When adding black to a pure hue it is called shade.
Tone – Adding gray to a pure hue is called tone.
Saturation – The measure of color and its intensity or strength.
Value – How light or dark a color is determines it value.
Color Theory

Color is the perceptual characteristic of light described by a color name. Specifically, color is light, and light is composed of many colors—those we see are the colors of the visual spectrum: red, orange, yellow, green, blue, and violet. Objects absorb certain wavelengths and reflect others back to the viewer. We perceive these reflected wavelengths as color. In essence it is the way we see color.

Color theory: in the visual arts is practical guidance to color mixing and the visual impacts of color combinations. A make-up artist should understand the Basics of Color Theory in order to know how colors work with each other, and how one color will influence another by placing it next to, on top of each other, or even how the color will result in when you mix them together.

As a make-up artist, you will always have clients ask you, "What colors look best on me?" or "How do I find the best foundation shade?"

To answer this question properly and give your clients the guidance they are looking for, you the professional makeup artist must have a clear understanding of basic color theory. And in order to make the right choice for your clients and create the best color scheme to compliment their desired look you will need to know how the color wheel works.

The Color Wheel

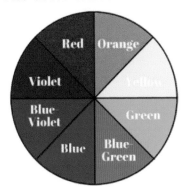

The color wheel: Consists of primary, secondary, and tertiary colors. It is a tool to help guide you visually.

Primary Colors: Are known as the fundamental colors, they cannot be created from a mixture. In a prism of sunlight these are the three main spectral colors seen: Yellow, red and blue. All colors are made from these three primary colors.

Secondary Colors: When you mix equal parts of two primary colors you will obtain a secondary color. There are only three secondary colors in the color wheel: Orange, green and violet.

Tertiary colors: (TUR-shee-ayr-ee) when mixing equal amounts of a primary color and secondary color you will achieve a tertiary color. These colors are always named after the primary color first and then secondary colors second. (Red-orange, yellow-orange, yellow-green, blue-green, blue-violet, red-violet)

Warm and Cool Tones

The basis to all color selection is in understanding warm and cool tones. The color wheel is broken into two parts: warm and cool tones. Having a strong understanding of the two is absolutely essential because all colors can have cool or warm tones.

WARM	COOL
WARM SHADES TO LOOK FOR:	COOL SHADES TO LOOK FOR.
PEACH	ROSY PINK
PEACHY PINK	BLUE
ORANGE	BLUE-GREEN
YELLOW	PURPLES/VIOLETS
ORANG-Y RED	DEEP, BLUE-BASED REDS

Warm Tones: Range from red red-orange trough gold to shades of yellows. Warm tones have yellow under tones.
Cool Tones: Dominated by blues, greens. All cool tones have a blue undertone.

All colors can be turned to warm or cool based on the amount of blue or red is added.
Example: If red is orange based then it is a warm red. If red is blue based then it is a cool red.

Complementary Colors

Are found directly across from each other on the color wheel. When complimentary colors are placed next to each other, each color will make the other look brighter resulting in greater contrast. Complimentary colors are the most flattering colors for your clients eye color and will be the best option for you as you begin applying makeup to clients. As you mature with your makeup skills you will feel more confident with color and how to can create stunning looks on your clients.

Understanding color theory as it applies to makeup is crucial to having a flawless look for your client and it is up to you to learn the rules to color as it applies to your makeup artistry techniques.

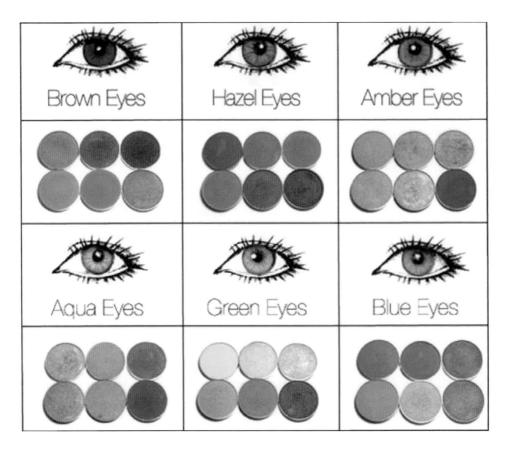

If your eyes are brown with a warm and yellowy glow, go directly across the color wheel and use shades of purples.

Example: If you have blue eyes go directly across the color wheel and use coppery orange shades.

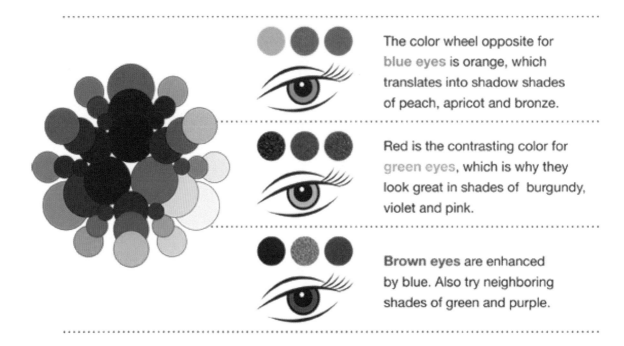

The color wheel opposite for blue eyes is orange, which translates into shadow shades of peach, apricot and bronze.

Red is the contrasting color for green eyes, which is why they look great in shades of burgundy, violet and pink.

Brown eyes are enhanced by blue. Also try neighboring shades of green and purple.

Choosing Blush

Many makeup artists make the mistake of using blush to contour and add shape to their client's faces, when in fact blush was designed to add life and color to the face. Blushes fall into two skin tone categories, ivory-beige or bronze-ebony. Rich, dark, warm blushes should be used on darker skin tones, bronze-ebony skin tones, while ash-light shades should be used on ivory-beige skin tones. There are a few shades that work on both warm and cool skin tones; these colors have apricot hues.

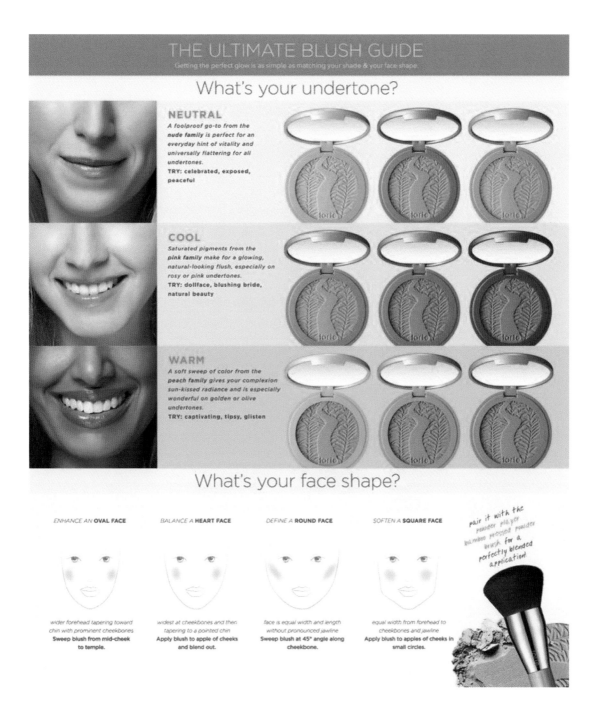

Choosing Lip Color

Choosing a lipstick or lip liner will directly depend on the size of your client's lips and their skin tone.

Ivory to beige skin tones: Use a bright colorful warm tones lip colors to make look youthful. Deep dark lip color will age this skin tone due to higher contrast and make lips look smaller.

Bronze to Ebony skin tones: Brown colors look very natural. They can get away with wearing bright colors as long as it's a warm tone.

If your client has small lips always use a lighter color so their lips look fuller, darker colors make lips look smaller.

Always choose lip colors that tend to fall on the warm side of the color wheel for best results.

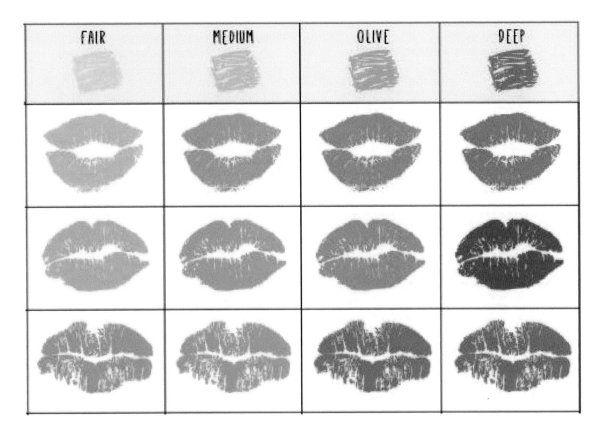

Determining Skin Tone

Picking the correct foundation color for your client should not be taken lightly. In the world of makeup artistry a flawless looks starts with a flawless base.

Undertones on your face and body differ from person to person; it is as individual as you are. So when it comes to foundation, you should try to match it as perfectly as you can to the undertone of your face, your jawline, your neck, and your chest. This is where it really matters when picking out a flawless foundation match.

So what is your skin tone? Some skin looks more yellow or has a yellow hue, other's pink or olive with a green hue, some will say they have a peachy undertone and dark skin tones might say they have a red undertone, but in general all skin tones fall into three categories, warm, cool and neutral. Warm skin tones tend to be more yellow, cool skin tones are pinker, while neutral skin tones have a mix of both colors. But what about olive skin tone? Well some say it counts as neutral a mixture of both blue and green, but you will need to look to see if your shade of green is more yellow or bluer.

Let's Determine Your Skin's Undertone

Warm: Yellow undertones, green veins, white clothing makes you look vibrant, and gold jewelry suits you best.

Cool: Pink undertones, blue veins, beige clothing makes you look vibrant, and silver jewelry suits you best.

Neutral: A mix of cool and warm undertones, white and beige make you look vibrant, gold and silver jewelry suit you, your skin tans but it can also burn.

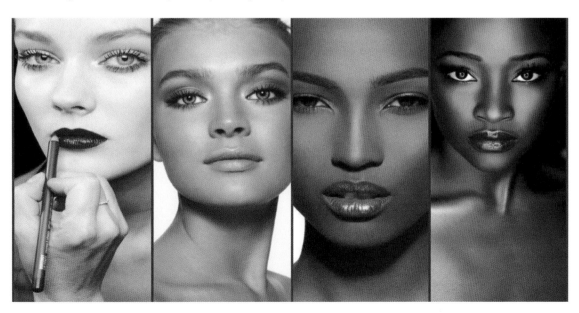

Let's Determine Your Ideal Foundation Shade

Undertones on you face and body can differ, but when it comes to foundation, you should match it to the undertone of your neck and chest.

Warm Undertone: Look for a foundation with a yellow hue and make sure to test it down your jawline and into your neck. If at all possible walk out into the natural light to determine that the color melds into your skin and be sure give it time to oxidize. You will know it's perfect when you can barely see it when you apply it, remember you are trying to match your skin color not change it.

Cool Undertone: Look for a foundation with a pink hue or ash hue and make sure to test it down your jawline and into your neck. If at all possible walk out into the natural light to determine that the color melds into your skin and be sure give it time to oxidize. You will know it's perfect when you can barely see it when you apply it, remember you are trying to match your skin color not change it.

Neutral Undertone: Look for a foundation that has a mixture of warm and cool or if you can't find this you may need to mix your colors to create the perfect match. Make sure to test it down your jawline and into your neck and if at all possible walk out into the natural light to determine that the color melds into your skin and be sure give it time to oxidize. You will know it's perfect when you can barely see it when you apply it, remember you are trying to match your skin color not change it.

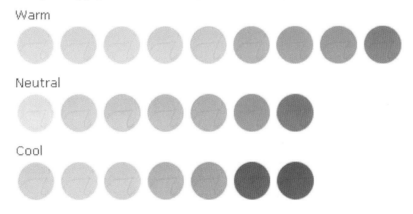

Foundation color matching is the most important piece of your daily makeup routine and should be a priority in your makeup choices.

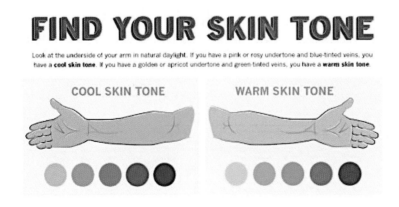

Facial Shapes & Features

"Knowing your face shape is the first step to creating your most beautiful look"
- Kevyn Aucoin

People have unique faces; they come in all shapes and sizes but for the most part here are the seven categories of the basic face shape: oval, square, round, triangle, heart, rectangle (oblong), and diamond. Every makeup artist should know the seven basic face shapes in order to be successful at enhancing your client's features.

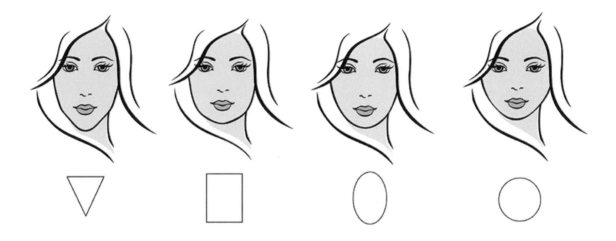

Oval: This face shape is considered the ideal face shape because it is not overly round or too full, it's well balanced and symmetrical. It is widest at the cheekbones and tapers in slightly at the forehead and jawline.

Round: Has a softly rounded jawline, a rounded hairline, short chin, it is widest at the cheekbones and it is usually not much longer than it is wide.

Square: This face shape is straight and angular, the width of the forehead, cheekbones, and jawline are equal.

Oblong/Rectangular: This face shape appears rectangular; the cheekbones are not much wider than the forehead and jawline. This shape has prominent cheekbones and has very similar qualities to a square face except it is longer.

Triangle: This face shape appears as an inverted triangle (upside down). It appears widest at the forehead and tapers down towards the jaw. The inverted triangle Is widest in the jawline and tapers in toward the forehead resembling a pear.

Heart: Having prominence in the cheekbones, the heart shape face is soft rather than angular. It starts as an inverted triangle, tapering out and up toward the cheekbones where it rounds out and closes off at the forehead, which is the widest part. People with heart-shaped faces usually have a widow's peak.

Diamond: The diamond shaped face is widest at the cheekbones and has a narrow forehead and chin appearing angular in form. The measurements of the hairline and jaw are about the same.

Eye Shapes

Eyes have been said to be the window to the soul, they can speak a thousand words with just one glance. As an aspiring makeup artist you must know all the basic eye shapes and have a thorough understanding of eye shapes to allow you to bring harmony and balance to facial features.

Round Eyes: Round shaped have more visible whites of the eyes and they appear large. This shape can sometimes be mistaken for protruding eyes.
When working on a client with round eyes you will want to elongate them, make them so they appear more almond shaped.

- Apply medium eye shadow to the eyelid up to the crease.
- Extend the shade to the outer eye corner and continue down along the lower eyelid.
- Use darker liner to line top and bottom eyelids. Extend eyeliner out and up beyond the eyelid in the outer corners.
- Apply mascara to the top lashes only, more on the outer half.
- Use darker eyeliner to line the outer two-thirds of both top and bottom eyelids or line only outer halves of the eyes and extend the line out and up in the outer corner.

Close-Set Eyes & Wide-Set Eyes
Close-set eyes fall really close to the bridge of the nose, while wide-set eyes sit apart from the bridge of the nose.

Corrective Applications for Close Set Eyes: The goal for corrective makeup when doing close-set eyes is to make them look evenly placed on the face. You can correct close-set eyes by putting a darker color of eye shadow in the outer corner of the eye and apply the mascara not only upward but also outward.

- Apply a pale eye shadow all over the lid up to the crease.
- Apply a dark shadow in the outer V and crease of the eye.
- Apply a light shadow on the inner corner of the eye.
- Apply mascara in an upward and outward.

Corrective applications for wide-set eyes: The goal for corrective makeup when doing wide-set eyes is to make them look evenly placed on the face and closer together. You can correct wide-set eyes by putting a darker color of eye shadow in the inner corner of the eye and apply the mascara not only upward but also inward.

- Apply a medium color eye shadow to the inner corner and floating lid of the eye towards the nose.
- Blend a light color shadow from the middle part of the eyelid out. This will shade the inner portion of the eye and highlight the outer portion of the eye, creating an illusion of balance. Make sure to blend the light color and dark color in the center of the eye so there is no line of demarcation.
- When applying eyeliner apply it all the way to the inside corner of the nose on the top and bottom of the eyelid.
- Apply mascara upward and inward.

Eyebrow Shapes

Proper eyebrow shaping will give you a polished look and enhance your client's appearance and it is your job as a makeup artist to learn the art of eyebrow shaping/arching. Defining eyebrows is it's own form of art and will take a lot of practice and maybe even advanced training.

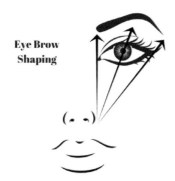

Lip Shapes

Lips come in all shapes and sizes from full and pouty to thin and lean. Your job as a makeup artist is to make them look more proportionate, falling directly under the nostrils with the appearance of curves or even peaks. As you practice on faces you will come across some clients where one side of their lip is different from the other. This is where you will need training and a good eye so it is important to have an understanding of how to enhance lip shapes to help your client have a harmonious face.

Small Thin Lips: Outline both the upper and lower lips. Fill in with soft or frosted colors to make them appear larger.

Large Full Lips: Draw a thin line just inside the natural lip line. Use soft, flat or dark lipstick colors that will make large lips look smaller.

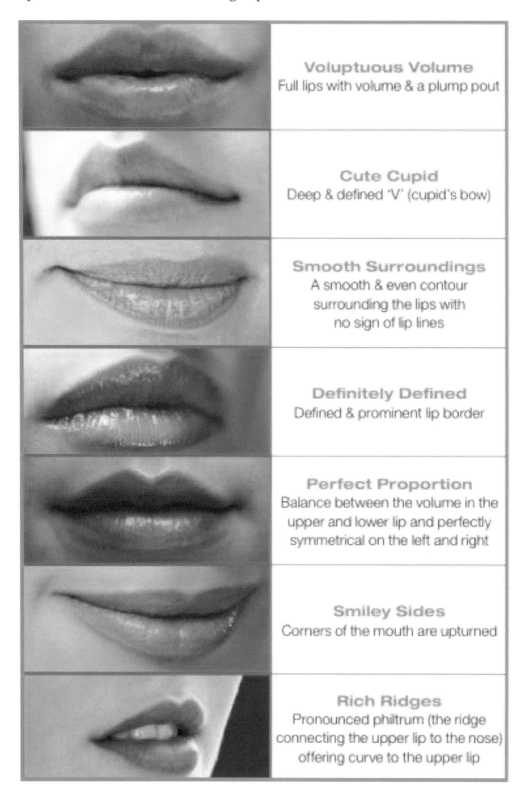

Voluptuous Volume
Full lips with volume & a plump pout

Cute Cupid
Deep & defined 'V' (cupid's bow)

Smooth Surroundings
A smooth & even contour surrounding the lips with no sign of lip lines

Definitely Defined
Defined & prominent lip border

Perfect Proportion
Balance between the volume in the upper and lower lip and perfectly symmetrical on the left and right

Smiley Sides
Corners of the mouth are upturned

Rich Ridges
Pronounced philtrum (the ridge connecting the upper lip to the nose) offering curve to the upper lip

Skin Type-Skincare-Makeup

Skin Type

Normal Skin: Normal skin has a healthy, flawless appearance. It looks matte and feels soft and smooth. It has the least skin problems and is less common than other types. Use a moisturizer for normal skin and toner without alcohol.

Combination Skin: Combination skin is usually of uniform color and plump looking. With this skin type there are oily areas on the nose, chin, and forehead, sometimes called the T-Zone. The care of this type of skin requires treating each zone separately with specific products. There are moisturizers formulated for combination skin, but results are better if you use two different products. To remove excess oil or grime, use an astringent facial toner. Use a matting product before applying foundation and hydrate the rest of the face with normal or dry skin cream.

Dry Skin: Most women use oil-based products to combat facial dryness but this is not the best approach because dry skin is actually lacking water. To keep dry skin hydrated, it is best to drink lots of water, use hyaluronic-based moisturizers, and apply water based moisturizing creams at least twice a day.

Oily Skin: Oily skin is usually plump, shiny and dewy to the touch. Use astringents for this type of skin to help absorb excess oil. Use water or gel based creams and avoid oil-based products so you don't over saturate the skin. With this type of skin, the onset of wrinkles is often delayed, pores may be visible and the sun is tolerated quite well.

Sensitive Skin: This skin type is easily irritated, leading to redness and spots. It can also appear scaly, especially around the eyebrows and nostrils. With sensitive skin, it's best to avoid the sun as it produces dryness and tightness, avoid sun exposure and any product containing alcohol. On sensitive skin, use hypoallergenic products or creams containing soothing ingredients such as chamomile or aloe vera. Rose water is a great product to use to calm the skin and keep it fresh.

What is your Skin Type?

After washing and cleaning, my skin is?

- Tight and a little stretched - Dry.
- Clean, but shiny within 20min - Oily.
- In good condition - Normal.
- Somewhat shiny in the "T" zone - Mixed.
- A little red and stings - Sensitive.

When I do not use creams, the next morning my skin is?

- Rough and scaly. - Dry.
- Greasy, shiny - Oily.
- Same as the previous day - Normal
- Somewhat shiny on the forehead - Mixed.
- Redness and scaling on cheeks or around nostrils - Sensitive.

The skin is a protective barrier against harmful agents such as bacteria, chemicals, and ultraviolet rays. Whatever your skin type there are three basic skincare rules to keep it youthful and healthy in appearance.

1. Clean it regularly and always remove all makeup.
2. Moisturize and care for your skin with products that suit your needs.
3. Protect your skin from external elements like the sun, smoke, wind, air conditioning etc. all these elements affect the condition of your skin.

Skincare

As part of your daily skin care and makeup removal routine, skin needs extra care to protect it from external factors and prevent signs of fatigue and premature aging.

Nourishing creams: these are not needed before the age of 30. Up to this age, the skin doesn't need extra lipids. For those over 30, we recommend applying a nourishing cream at night, as some active ingredients can be damaging if exposed to the sun.

Eye creams and lip contour products: these are specific products for the treatment of sagging, dehydration, and wrinkles in the sensitive areas around the eyes and lips.

Serum: serum is a concentrated, high-value cosmetic with a specific action. It may be a firming serum, moisturizer, or anti-aging product. It has a smooth texture, is absorbed very quickly, and penetrates deep into the skin. It doesn't replace a moisturizer but complements it.

Sunscreen: this protects the skin from UVA rays that cause skin aging and can cause skin cancer and also from UVB rays, which create redness, sunburn and a predisposition to skin cancer.

Scrubs: these are creams that help to remove dead skin cells. There is two types: fine for sensitive and normal skin and coarse for oily or combination skin.

Masks: in general, masks play an important role in penetrating through the layers of the skin to nourish, cleanse, and smooth in a deep and effective way. They come in weekly and monthly applications. They're not designed for daily use, as their high concentration of active ingredients could be harmful if used too often.

Specific cosmetic treatments: the usual treatment program for facial cleansing comprises of, makeup removal, exfoliation, pore extraction, facial massage and a facial mask, this is recommended once a month as a basic cosmetic treatment.

Medical dermatological treatments: make up artistry works best on healthy skin. If you're requested to makeup a client who has skin problems it's best to refer her/him to a dermatologist.

Makeup

The cosmetic industry is filled with many different brands of makeup. There is a specialty makeup out there designed for just about everything from brow kits to lip stains. This can be very overwhelming when you're just starting out so let's break it up into sections so you can get a better understanding of all the different types of makeup.

Foundation

Known as base makeup foundation comes in all skin tone shades and is applied all over the face including the neck and down into the décolleté. Foundation is the secret to an even, flawless finish. There are several different types of foundation and come in three forms.

Liquid Foundation: Comes in pretty little glass jars or tubes and gives an all over dewy finish. Liquid foundation can be applied with a disposable makeup sponge, and can be used under powder to help powder adhere to the skin.

Cream Foundation: A heavier form of liquid foundation that usually comes in a compact and is applied with fingertips and a beauty blender. This heavier and thicker foundation is used to cover skin issues and scars.

Powder Foundation: Which comes in compact containers gives an all over even matte finish and is usually applied with a powder brush.

Eye Shadows

Help to give the eyes definition and there are thousands of shades and colors to choose from and they come in many different forms. No matter what form you decide to use remember to look for high pigment content and smooth application.

Loose Pigments: Pure pigments designed to work loose and as a makeup artist this type of shadow is easy to use and can give great coverage and depth with very little application. These are usually found in small containers and are used dry or mixed with a makeup medium for a more vibrant look.

Shadow Palette: The eye shadow palette is most familiar to us, we see it everywhere and most of us have used this type of eye shadow most of our adult lives. Shadow palettes range in size and pigment content and usually contain complimentary colors designed to work well with each other in the eye shadow application. When using eye shadow palettes try to ensure the product is highly pigmented and goes on smoothly.

Cream Shadow: This eye shadow is fairly new on the mainstream market and is designed with a creamy consistency; it goes on smooth and usually dries quickly to give great coverage. Learning to use cream shadows takes practice and will require that you the makeup artist pick the products that last all day and don't crease on the eyelid.

Liners

Eye Liner: Will easily become your best friend when you find the one you love. Eyeliner is a tool to help frame the eyes and when used correctly you can make your clients face look more dramatic and enhance their eye shape. Eyeliner was designed to define the eye like no other makeup can and like all the other types of makeup; eyeliner comes in many different colors and consistencies.

Pencil Liner: Pencil eyeliners can be creamy waxy or same where in between. When using a pencil liner you draw it on the eyelids right above the lash line. The tip of the pencil should be touching the lash line at all times to create an even look.

Liquid Liner: Comes in a bottle with a twist off cap and usually has a very thin brush at the end. Liquid eyeliner takes a lot of practice and it can get very messy if you don't have a steady hand. Unlike a pencil liner, it is painted on and needs a few seconds to dry.

Mascara: Comes in many different colors but the most common colors are Black, Brown and Blue. Mascara is used to lengthen, strengthen, curl, thicken and separate the lashes. The ultimate objective is to enhance the lashes to their fullest. Every makeup kit should contain mascara and in the three most popular shades. With experience you will find the mascara you prefer and which type of disposable applicator works best for you.

Blush: Blush brings warmth and liveliness to the face. It is used to give the face the final glow. Coming in a variety of containers and consistencies the most popular kind of blush is pressed powder.

Lipstick: The purpose of lipstick is to enhance the lips, balance them out to achieve proportion, and bring all the elements of the face together.

No matter what type of makeup you choose be sure to choose quality over quantity.

Correct & Conceal

Concealers are the secret of the Universe as Bobbi Brown would say and while concealers are available that can cover tattoos, spots, blemishes, scars, redness, and bruises, most makeup artists use concealer to lighten dark circles under the eyes and brighten the face. Concealers and correctors are formulated for different uses and should be used according to their design. Pick a concealer and, when needed, a corrector designed for each of your client's problem areas.

Correctors were designed to cover tattoos, spots, blemishes, scars, redness, and bruises and severe under eye darkness but most people use a concealer to lighten dark circles under the eyes and brighten the face.

Concealers and correctors are formulated differently and are designed for each specific use. Pick a concealer and when needed a corrector designed for each of your problem areas. Under-eyes concealers are not formulated for use on blemishes or areas of redness this is when you need a corrector. Concealers are creamier in consistency and lighter than the skin tone. Using under eye concealer on areas of redness will only highlight the imperfections. The yellow-toned foundation that matches the skin tone is the best way to adequately cover blemishes, scars and tattoos.

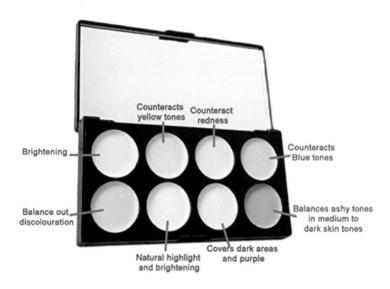

Correctors are available for extreme under-eye darkness. When a regular concealer cannot fully lighten the under eye area, a peach or pink corrector is used to counter balance the purple or green tone. A regular yellow toned concealer is usually lightly layered over the corrector to lighten the under eye area. Occasionally, those with extremely deep purple or green coloration under the eye will not need the layer of regular concealer.

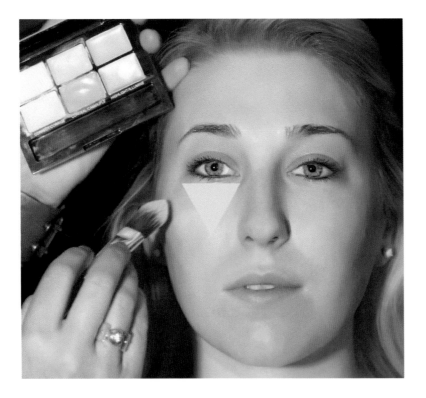

Corrector Application

Determine the areas on the face, neck and chest that need to be concealed and choose the correct color to be applied to those areas.

Do the corrector steps before you apply foundation.

1. Apply a small amount of corrector in the right shade to hide a flaw and
2. Tap it lightly on to the area.
3. Blend the outer edges in a feathering technique to blend in to the skin.
4. Wait until product is dry before applying foundation.

Concealer application

The application of under eye concealer is the most important step in any makeup routine. Concealer is the one product that, when chosen and applied correctly, can instantly lift and brighten the face.

Concealer steps after you apply foundation.

1. Choose a color that is one shade lighter than the foundation.
2. Apply in a V shape below the eye and blend in upward strokes.
3. Use a sponge blender to blend out the edges for a seamless look.

Contouring & Highlighting

Contouring and Highlighting
When it comes to highlighting and contouring, there's a fine line between enhancing your best features and changing the shape of your face. With contouring and highlighting we can bring out the cheekbones, slim the nose, and subtly sculpt the face while at the same time maintain your clients best features.

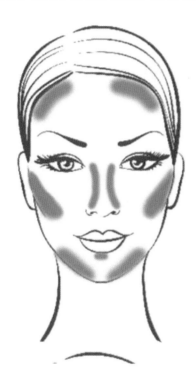 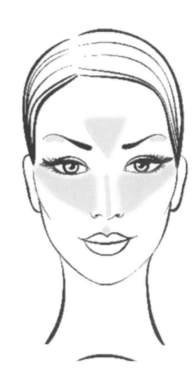

Contour Technique
Old school contouring used to mean layers of dark dramatic makeup with harsh angles. The twenty-first century version is all about enhancing cheekbones, slimming your clients face, and tricking the eye in a believable way.

Use the Right Products
You only need two products, a matte contouring cream or powder and a highlighter. Try contouring with a cream, you can pat it on with your fingertips and it has a natural finish that doesn't look like makeup. If you're more comfortable with powder, choose a sheer formula, which gives a softer contour.

While the formula you use is up to you, make sure you're consistent. That means using all cream or all powder products. Layering different textures can cause a caked effect, and it won't blend as seamlessly. You are the artist so be very cautious so that your application looks fresh and seamless.

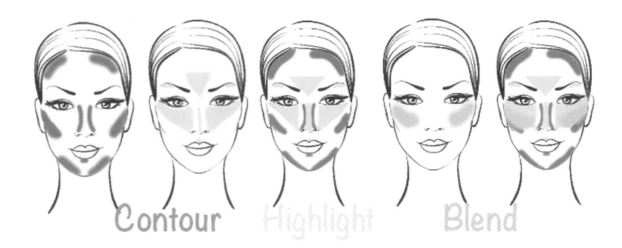

Consider Skin Tone

Anything that stands out too much against the skin is going to look obvious. If your client is fair, use a contouring cream or powder that's one shade darker than their skin tone. In keeping with the idea of shadows, look for formulas with a neutral cast and stay away from anything too red or orange, like most bronzers. Bronzers are for bronzing and a sun kissed look, they are not the ideal product to use for contouring the face. Your finished result should look as natural as possible.

Natural Highlighting

Highlighter should be almost the color of your skin, with just a hint of shimmer or reflection, avoid anything with sparkles or glitter, which can look chalky or just plain unnatural. Remember the key is good coverage with a natural looking end result.

Use the Right Tools

Creams: Use your fingers, they warm the makeup so it melts and blends more seamlessly into your clients skin.

Powder: Use a fan brush, which has natural bristles. There are few bristles, they're soft and you are less likely to overdo it. The shape of the brush lets you really control the placement.

Specific Shading

To give the appearance of cheekbones have your client suck in their cheeks, it's the best way to find the hollows under the cheek. Then, working from the hairline inward, shade along (and just beneath) the sunken area, stop about an inch from the corner of your clients mouth, then blend well with your finger or a sponge. To slim your clients nose, blend two lines of the contour cream or powder from the start of their brows down the sides of the bridge of the nose with a small shadow brush. Then blend well downward to give the illusion of a slimmer nose.

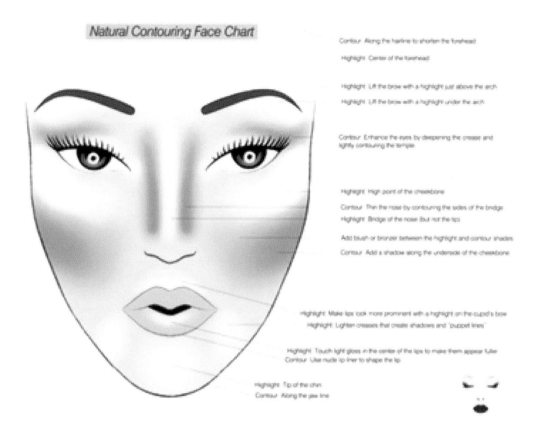

BE STRATEGIC

Highlighting is especially important when you're contouring because it brings the light back into your face, but once again, you don't want to overdo it. Lightly dust or blend highlighter above your client's cheekbone, down the top of your client's nose, and then dab a small amount on the brow bone under the brow, on the center of their chin and just one tap on the tip of cupids bow above the lip.

UNDERSTAND FACE SHAPES

Not all of the rules of highlighting and contouring are universal; it's also important to keep your clients face shape in mind. If they have a round face, contouring under their cheekbones can make it appear smaller. If they have a narrow face, it could make it look even longer. Take the safe approach and shade along the top of the forehead and a bit on the chin. This technique softens angular features and creates a more rounded effect. The goal is to use your products strategically giving the illusion of the perfect oval face shape. Contouring and highlighting is all about shadows and light and using products to enhance the face to get optimal results for your client.

BLENDING

Blending can be the most important step in the contouring and highlighting, even if you've gone overboard, blending with a sponge, brush or even your fingers can fix to much product application. If you use powder products run a fluffy brush with natural fibers over the finished look in a circular buffing motion. Hold your brush softly with your hand toward the end of the handle giving your products a softer, more seamless finish.

BLUSH

Try to be very careful when adding your blush product. Adding a bright blush could give you that retro stripe and make your client look out of date. In turn leaving your client's cheeks completely colorless can have a flattening and colorless effect. Stick with colors that flatter like a soft peach or pink if they have fair skin, or soft plum for darker complexions. Blend a cream formula on the apples of your client's cheeks for a natural flush look. Blush is made only for the cheeks.

Contouring is a skill that will require hours of practice working with cream and powder products. Take advantage of your friends and family members and practice the art of contouring and highlighting to become proficient at the skill of understanding shadows and light and how it relates to the face. Face sculpting for everyday makeup should be subtle and well blended. Face sculpting for stage or fantasy makeup will require a heavy hand with less blending to create a face sculpt that is obvious and enhanced. As a makeup artist it is up to you to know and understand the right time and place for heavy contouring and highlighting.

Highlighting is a fun way to add light and shimmer to the face but remember leave the heavy highlighting for the runway makeup, stage makeup, and editorial makeup you will be doing in the near future.

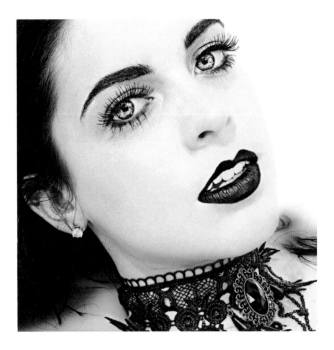

Shadowing the Eye

Shadowing the eyes is the most challenging application of the entire makeup application but if you follow these easy to apply steps you will master the technique very quickly. As a makeup artist you will be asked to do many different eye looks but this is the basic application where every eye look begins.

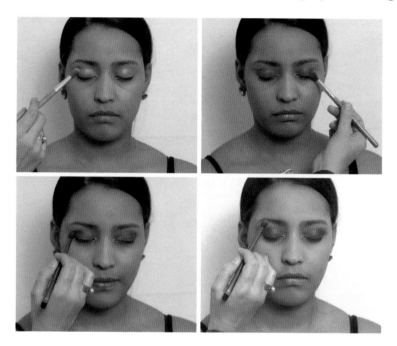

Shadowing Steps

1. Apply primer to the eyelids.
2. Apply light beige to the entire eyelid.
3. Apply a pink or peach to the floating lid stopping at the crease line.
4. Apply a charcoal or dark brown to the outer corner of the lower lid in the crease line, blending 1/3 of the way toward the center and then to the lash line 1/3 of the way in.
5. Blend well.
6. Apply shimmer beige or light silver to the inner corner of the lower lid and just below the brow on the brow bone.
7. Blend well.

The secret to great eye shadow application is using quality products with a high pigment content, using quality brushes, and blending well to get a seamless look of each color coming together. Do not leave any harsh lines of demarcation.

Showcasing the eyes is important, you want the eyes to look alluring and attractive, but try not to overdo the look, keep it simple and flawless.

Lining the Eye

A world without eyeliner is like brunch without mimosas, and since we'd never wish either situation on even our worst enemy, we will explore one of our all time favorite beauty essentials. Eyeliner is and always will be the most effective way to enhance the eyes. Pencil, gel or liquid; winged, smudged or clean; the options are plentiful, so let's break it down and explore all your eye lining options.

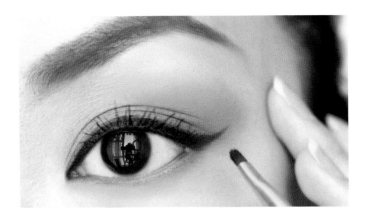

Pencil Eyeliner

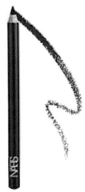

A basic eye pencil should be a makeup bag staple of every makeup artist. Pencils are quick and easy to work with and they're the gold standard when it comes to versatility. Use pencil eyeliner to add definition to the top and bottom lash lines, to line the waterline, or smudge it out to create a dramatic smoky eye. Use a pencil to get as close to the lash line as possible, make sure your pencil is always sharpened to a fine point. Look for a high-pigment pencil that is soft enough that it will not tug the skin yet long lasting to stay on all day. For the smoothest application, start by warming the tip of the pencil between your fingers and apply in short strokes across the eye. The pencil will always be your go to product and a must have in your beauty kit.

Cream and Gel Eyeliner

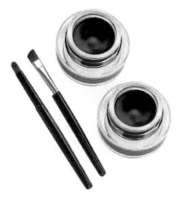

Creams and gels are a great alternative to liquid liner. They can be used to create the same precise lines, but the formulas are thicker allowing for an application that is more forgiving of shaky hands. Use potted cream and gel eyeliners with an angled brush to craft your cat eye or choose a smaller precision brush to create an ultra thin line. Cream and gel formulas are also ideal for tight-lining the waterline because an eyeliner brush can really push the color into the base of the lashes. Whether you go defined and precise or smudged and smoky remember to choose a longwearing formula and set it by pressing eye shadow on top of the liner to ensure its staying power.

Liquid Eyeliner

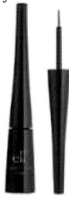

The coveted winged eyeliner look can be achieved by using any of the options above, but for the cleanest, most precise line, liquid liner is a must. Liquids tend to be the favorite of women with hooded eyelids and oily skin because although wet when applying the product, once dry they won't budge. With that in mind, keep pointed Q-tips handy to clean up mistakes as you go. With liquids you can choose a formula that dries to a matte finish or a patent leather-like gloss. Look for a product with a small, thin brush or applicator that will give you the most control, allowing you to create subtle definition as well as bolder lines. If you want a thicker line, apply more pressure to the brush or build up the line by layering your strokes.

Makeup Application

The 10 Step Makeup Application

The School of Makeup Artistry founder and master educator Toni Thomas designed the 10-step makeup application to make your job as a makeup artist easy and efficient. After working with clients and students for many years she realized that many women are confused about the process of applying makeup and the correct order in which we should apply our cosmetics. As a makeup artist if you are doing a full face of makeup on your client this is the application technique we recommend to achieve long lasting and flawless coverage for your clients.

1. Prime
Apply primer to the entire face and eye area.

Primer is the bond that creates a flawless finish for your makeup application to sit upon and get the lasting results you need for a long wearing makeup application.

2. Correct
Correct any skin discolorations using the color wheel as a guide. Correct blemishes, under eye discoloration, hyper pigmentation or facial features that need adjustments. This step is crucial in your makeup application so be sure to correct using your small concealer brush or a disposable applicator.

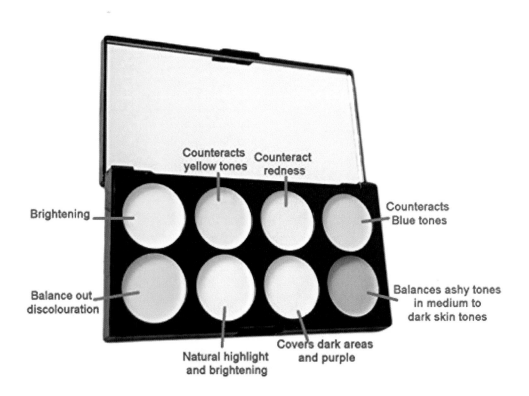

3. Foundation

Color Match
1. Apply a stripe of foundation from cheek down to the neck with a disposable applicator or your finger.
2. Choose the color that matches the skin so closely that it almost disappears into the skin.
3. Using your foundation brush in a sweeping motion, sweep the foundation in a upward and outward motion covering the entire face. You should always follow the direction of hair growth and blend the product till it looks flawless.

4.Conceal & Brighten

1. Start with a beige or yellow concealer one shade lighter than your skin tone.
2. Apply under the eyes and create a V-shape that runs from under your eye down to the top of your cheek and blend it with upward and outward strokes to the outer corner of your eye.

The finished look should appear well blended with no lines of demarcation.

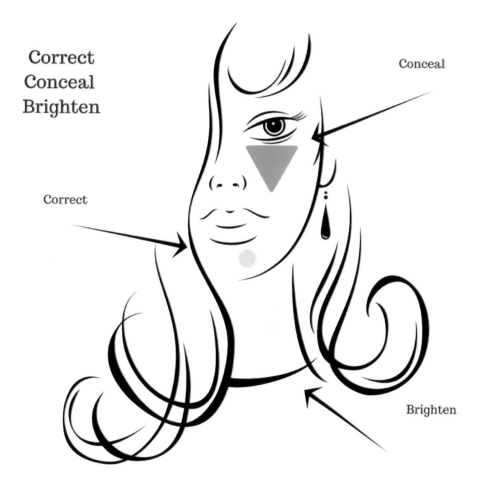

5.Set

Setting your concealer and foundation is an important step in your makeup application and one you don't want to miss. Use a quality translucent powder or a yellow toned translucent powder on the face and neck to give a shine free look that will ensure you have a perfect finish. Make sure to use a large fluffy powder brush.

1. Apply a quality setting powder in translucent or yellow-toned shade.
2. Sparingly apply the setting powder to the full face and neck.
3. Do not over apply this product or it will look caked.

If you are working on a more mature client, we suggest not using any powder it tends to settle in fine lines. Wait to set the product with setting spray.

6. Contour & Bronze

Your contour color should be one shade darker than the natural skin tone but not to dark that it will make a face look over sculpted and un-natural.

1. Use a contour shade just a bit darker than the skin tone and apply just below each cheekbone, sweeping out toward the hair.
2. If necessary on a large forehead contour along the hairline to slim the face.
3. Slim down a large chin by placing a fine dust of contour under the chin enhancing the end of the chin bone.
4. If you feel like you need to slim down the nose apply along the top sides of the nose and blend downward to give the illusion of a slimmer nose.

There is no need to contour rich or dark olive skin tones they are blessed with rich skin that needs no contouring. We will talk further on how you can give depth to rich skin tone by using cream highlighters and light concealers.

Bronzing

1. Apply bronzer just above the contour and blend well.
2. Apply to the chest area if you're client is wearing a strapless or low cut top.
3. Bronzer can also be applied to the forehead and on the cheeks or anywhere that the sunlight would hit on the face or anywhere that needs a kiss of sun.
4. Don't overdo bronzer it can quickly darken the face appearing dirty.

7. Blush

For a fresh and luminous glow use a two-step blush application. Blush when applied correctly wakes the face up and adds warmth.

1. Apply a light natural shade of blush to the cheekbones moving in an upward swirl to the hairline.

2. Next apply a brighter pink or peach shade and apply just to the apples of the cheek then lightly blended into the natural shade to bring the two colors together. This will brighten your clients face for a realistic blush finish.

8. Eyes

Showcasing the eyes is the most challenging application of the makeup application but if you follow these easy to apply steps you will master the technique very quickly.

Eye Shadowing Steps

1. Apply primer to the eyelids.
2. Apply light beige in shimmer or matte to the entire eyelid.
3. Apply a pink, peach or taupe to the middle of the lid stopping at the crease line.
4. Apply a charcoal or dark brown to the outer corner of the lid in the crease line, blending 1/3 of the way toward the center and then to the lash line 1/3 of the way in. Blend well.
5. Apply a beige or light highlighter color to the inner corner of the lower lid and just below the brow on the brow bone. Use this color to lightly blend all other colors together

The secret to great eye shadow application is using quality products with high pigment content, and blending well to get a seamless look of each color coming together. Showcasing the eyes is important, you want the eyes to look full and well accentuated on the face.

Eye Shadow Order

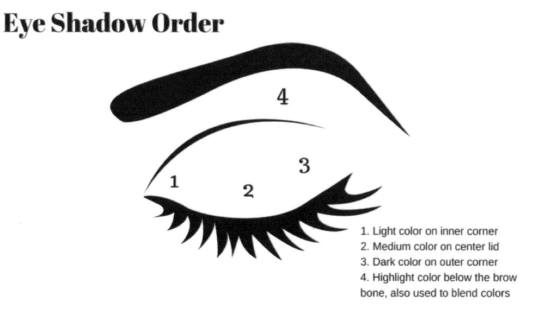

1. Light color on inner corner
2. Medium color on center lid
3. Dark color on outer corner
4. Highlight color below the brow bone, also used to blend colors

Eye Liner

Eyeliner doesn't have to be difficult even if it can be challenging at first to understand how to hold your brush and how to get a smooth line but with practice and quality brushes eye lining can be easy to achieve.

Try the tight-lining technique for your eyeliner to showcase the eyes; this technique is much easier to apply with damp eye shadow using a liner brush or very small stiff flat brush. Don't be afraid to test out liner products. This technique can be done with powder shadows, liner pencil or lose pigments.

1. Line the upper lash line with a dark charcoal, dark brown or rich black.
2. Line the lower lash line with the same color coming in only 3/4 of the way.
3. Soften the liner by smudging it with a bigger flat brush.

Eye lining is a skill that requires a lot of practice, use a black eye shadow and dampen your brush to create a thick paste then apply the paste with a fine lining brush to the upper lash line and the lower lash line and to the upper inside lash line. You can darken the look be adding a gel liner over the top of the upper lash line when you have completed your entire eye makeup application

Brows

Defining the eyebrows will create a natural frame for the face and makes the eyes of your client pop. Be sure to use the correct color brow powder or brow pencil to fill-in brows, we suggest a two-color brow process to get a natural look.

1. Apply the first color the same as your natural brow color or hair color to the lower brow line and move in hair like strokes to the out brow
2. Use the lighter color to the inside corner of the brow using hair like strokes and to the upper hairline to give the brow depth and definition.

Brows complete the face and without some type of enhancement or correction you can leave your clients face looking unfinished if you skip this step. Brow products come in pencils, powders and even gels.

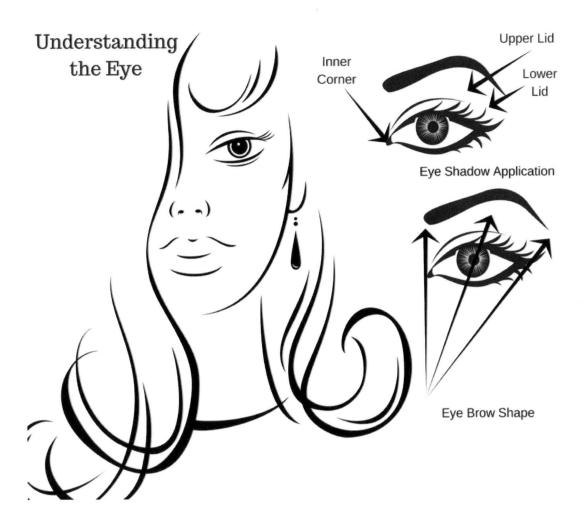

Eyebrow Shaping

Eyebrow shaping is a skill you will develop over time but the basic shape is as follows:

1. The brow starts on the inner corner of the nose. Use a thin long brush or your eyebrow pencil to gage the starting point of the brow. Place a small dot for you to start your brow line.
2. The arch of the brow should can be determined by holding your brow pencil at an angle coming up from the nose and running through the pupil o the eye. Place a small dot to gage where the high point of the brow should be.
3. The outer corner of the brow can be determined by placing the brow pencil at a wide angle coming from the corner of the nose and running on the outer corner of the eye. Place a small dot the gage where the eyebrow should finish.
4. Fill in the brow with small hair like strokes.

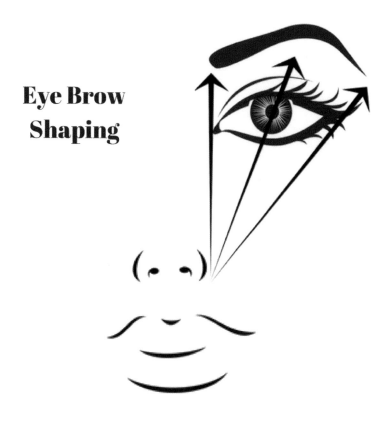

**Eye Brow
Shaping**

Lash Enhancements

Eyelashes open up and emphasize the eyes. Most lashes are transformed with a sweep of mascara and the use of an eyelash curler. Black mascara is usually a first choice for most women but women with very fair coloring or those who are naturally blonde should choose a lighter shade to make their eyes look fuller.

Mascara is a must for everyone but for those looking for something a bit more dramatic or for a special occasion false lashes are a good choice.

False eyelashes are used to create a more dramatic looking eye and for special effects for a very dramatic eye. Lashes can be applied individually, in a small section, or in a full band.

For those with sparse eyelashes, try smudging dark shadow at the lash line with a liner brush and then applying two thin coats of mascara.

When lashes have been lost due to alopecia or chemotherapy, a double application of powder shadow in a smoky shade helps create the illusion of lashes.

1. Apply powder shadow to line the lid keeping close to the lash line.
2. Then smudge the dry shadow from the lashes upward with a liner brush.

Alternatives

Not everyone is comfortable with eyelash extensions; this can be the case with a person who rarely wears makeup or someone who has never worn false lashes before. You may also have a client who prefers not to wear glue near her eyes or is allergic to the glues that are used with a false eyelash enhancement. But with the emerging advances in makeup today we have an alternative.

Fiber Lash Mascara

These new mascaras have a three-step process to get the same fullness and length that falsies give. These mascaras use a transplanting gel and fibers to get the same effect as today's eyelash extensions and false lashes.
There are many fiber mascaras on the market today and not all are created equal, make sure your fiber lash mascara is using an organic fiber as their fiber base and that there transplanting gel is of high quality.

Fiber Lash Mascara Application

Doing one eye at a time follow the recommended steps below
Step 1. Apply Transplanting Gel to the entire upper lash
Step 2. Quickly apply the fibers to the tips of the upper lash with a sweeping upward motion
Step 3. Apply a second coat of the Transplanting Gel to the tips of the upper lashes in a long sweeping motion to seal in the fibers and get the desired length.
Step 4. (Optional) Comb through the lashes with a metal-toothed lash comb to separate any stuck together lashes.
Step 5. Apply the transplanting gel to the lower lashes to desired look and length.
Repeat on other eye

False Lashes

If your client wants more pop, the easiest false lash technique for a novice is to use individual lashes that come with three lashes on each band. These lashes can be applied to the outer 1/3 corner of your lash line after your mascara application. This is so much easier than learning to apply false lashes which can be a challenge for even the most qualified makeup artist. The last thing you want to happen is to have a clients lash strip come loose, this will mean pulling off both lash stripes leaving you without the long lush lashes you desire. You can get these individual lashes at any beauty supply store and even at high-end retailers. Be sure to get the black glue used to apply the lashes so you don't have white dots on your lash line from the glue.

Individual Lash Application

Step 1: Choose the length of lash you want to use and trim the inner corner.
Step 2: Apply the lash glue to the end of the lash.
Step 3: Wait one minute to let the glue get tacky.
Step 4: Apply the lash onto your lash line.
Step 5: Set the lash by pushing down on the tip of the lash until it sets.
Step 6: Apply the lashes to just the 1/3 outer corner of your lash line.
Step 7: Wait a few minutes for the lashes to firm up and dry into place.

Lash Strip Application

Step 1: Choose the length of lash you want to use and trim if needed.
Step 2: Apply the lash glue to the strip end of the lash.
Step 3: Wait one minute to let the glue setup.
Step 4: Apply the lash onto your lash line.
Step 5: Set the lash by pushing down on the tip of the lash until it sets.
Step 6: Wait a few minutes for the lashes to firm up and dry into place.

9. Lips

Lip sculpting has become the newest rage in makeup and although we do not recommend trend makeup in the makeup application process we do think using this technique is a great way to give full lips. Achieving flawless lips is all about creating a plump and pouty look for a more romantic appearance to bring the lips forward. Lip products will be the first makeup to disappear during the day so using our three step application will ensure a longer lasting look, but even with that said, make sure you have your client has lip color on hand to refresh their look throughout the day.

Lip Sculpting

1. Line the lips with a color one shade darker than their natural lip color.
2. Line the corners of the lips one third of the way in with the liner color.
3. Fill in the area inside the lip liner with a shade that is exactly the same color as your client's natural lips with a lip liner pencil or lip stain.
4. Top off the lips with a lipstick in pink, peach or plum or use your favorite lip-gloss in a bright shade that makes the lip stand out.
5. Natural lips with a pop of color are the secret to lip sculpting.

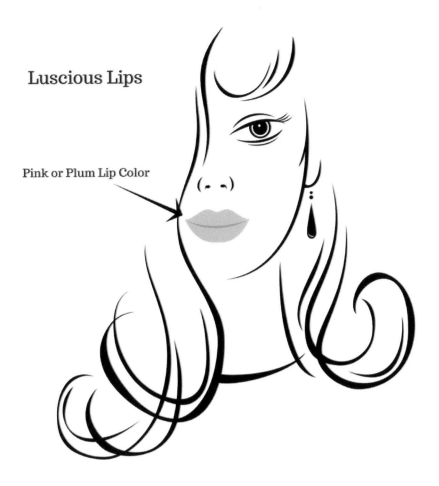

Luscious Lips

Pink or Plum Lip Color

10. Highlight & Set

Highlight

Highlighting in a makeup application is a relatively new concept in the world of makeup but it has been a well-kept secret of professionals, makeup artists have been highlighting their clients for years and understand the importance of this step in the makeup application. Makeup artists use highlighting to create light on the face and to brighten up a flawless makeup application.

Highlighting your clients face at the end of your makeup application gives it a shimmering glamorous glow with the illusion of perfect lighting.

1. Apply a powder highlighter below the brow, on the top of the brow bone, and on the top of the cheekbone just above the blush and under the corner of the eye.
2. Apply your powder highlighter to the cupids bow on the top of your upper lip.
3. Apply highlighter to the tip and top of the nose.
4. Apply the highlighter just above the brows if needed.

Set

The final step in any professional makeup application is setting the look and advising your client how best to keep the look fresh throughout the day and into the evening.

1. Apply a setting spray to your completed makeup application
2. Consult with your client about the importance of freshening up her lipstick throughout the day and keeping her skin hydrated. Well-hydrated skin keeps the face from looking sallow and dark.

Pro Makeup Application Before & After

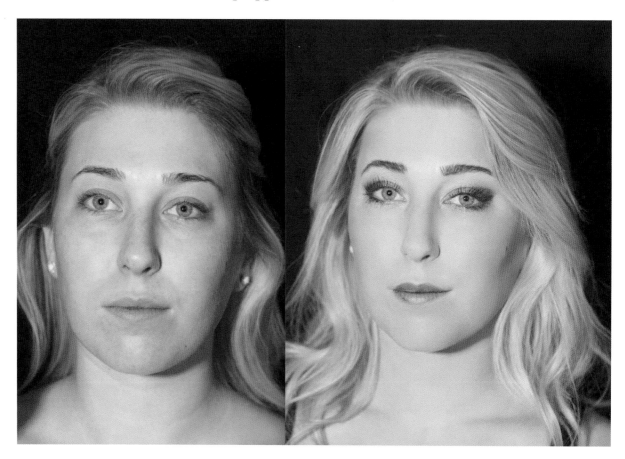

Evening Makeup

A Night Out

Just as you applied the basic daytime look for your client you will use the same skills you have learned in the previous module. You will color match the skin and color match the eye makeup and utilize all of your new color matching skills with each area of the face.

The night is for a more dramatic look and the day look can easily be transformed into a night look. Dramatic does not mean over done, it just means more intensity with a little flair to show off your client's personality.

Procedure:

1. With a dark gray, dark brown or black eyeliner or shadow, encircle the whole eye.
2. Smudge using a small shadow brush or disposable applicator.
3. With your shadow brush apply dark shadow from the upper lash line to the crease and make sure you are blending as you approach the crease.
4. Choose a darker eye shadow to shade the crease, apply this shadow (matte or shimmery) from the outer corner to the inner corner of the crease.
5. Blend the eye shadow in a wedge shape outward toward the brow. The shadow should be thickest near the eye, and taper out toward the tail of the brow.
6. Carefully blend applied shadow to the bottom lash line making sure you have no hard edges.
7. Highlight the brow bone with a shimmery neutral tone with a disposable eye shadow applicator.
8. Apply 3 heavy coats of mascara to the top lashes and 1 coat to the bottom lashes.

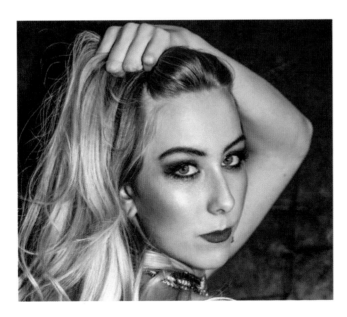

The Smoky Eye

The smoky eye is a soft, sultry and sexy makeup application. And without a doubt will be the number one requested service from you the Makeup Artist. To avoid a raccoon look the smoky eye application requires attention to detail and careful selection of color. It is the most common eye application requested for an evening look.

Smoky eyes can be made subtler by using less pigment or by choosing a dark to medium brown pigment as opposed to a black pigment. The can be more vibrant with more layering of color.

Procedure:
- Apply beige or gold shadow to the base of the eyelid and under the eye
- Apply gray shadow along crease to the outer corner of the lid extending slightly beyond the outer corner of the eye.
- Add black or dark brown eye shadow to the crease and outer corner of the eye
- Apply black liner in a thin line along the upper lash line. Gently smudge with a brush.
- Apply gray eye shadow along the lower lash line
- Apply black eye shadow along the outer corner of the lower lash line with your liner brush.
- Apply white shadow to the entire inner corner of the eye
- Apply white shadow beneath the brow
- Line the eyes with dark charcoal or black liner, smudge out and you are finished.

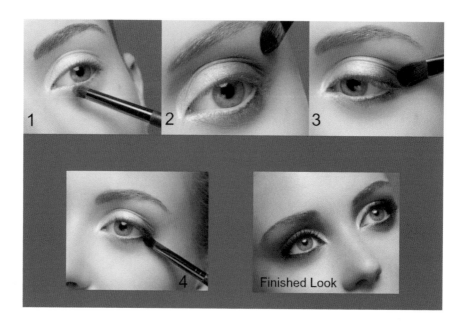

Bridal Makeup

As an Instructor the number one question I get when students arrive for their first day of master makeup class is when will we be doing bridal makeup? I think the stress of the perfect bridal look is a main concern for any makeup artist.

"The beauty of a woman must be seen from in her eyes, because that is the doorway to her heart, the place where love resides"
Audrey Hepburn

Bridal Skin Care

If your bridal client hasn't been diligent about her skincare now is the time for her to be getting regular facials, this will make a big difference in your client's skin and will help you to have the best base for your makeup application. It is up to you to help her find a skincare specialist and to guide her in proper skincare. Remind your client to prevent any last-minute irritation; she should skip extractions during her facial the month prior to her wedding.

A bride's makeup should be as natural looking as possible, but also emphasize her features so she looks flawless in photographs. Applying bridal makeup depends on both the theme and time of the wedding. An evening wedding can be slightly more dramatic with sultry eyes and bold shadows. Daytime bridal makeup should be minimal with neutral eye shadows and rosy lips. Every bride should emphasize blush and lips for the most foolproof and timeless bridal beauty.

No matter what a bride's style is, you should always apply makeup before putting on the wedding gown unless it must go over the head. In this case, use a cover to protect her precious wedding gown.

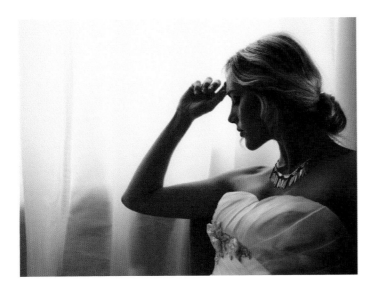

Step 1: Prime

Once your client's face is cleansed and moisturized use a quality primer that is lightweight one that will stabilize the products and keep the makeup in place all day. Your primer should and reduce the appearance of fine lines, large pores and mini-flaws of the face.

1. Apply primer with fingertips to the face and the lids of the eyes.
2. Wait three minutes for primer to set before applying makeup products.

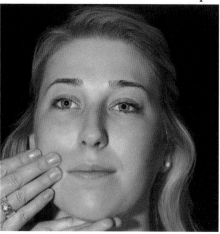

Step 2: Conceal, Correct & Brighten

Concealing is your bridal makeup secret weapon.

1. Start with a beige or yellow toned concealer under the eyes to hide dark circles and brighten the face.
2. Check the face for those little flaws you might want to conceal and use a pink or peach-toned corrector to neutralize discoloration or a green concealer to hide redness from rosacea and acne.
3. Brighten the neck and chest with a light bronzer and add a shimmer of highlighter.

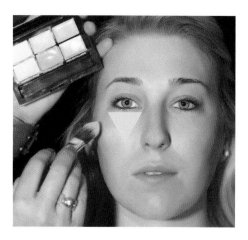

Step 3: Foundation

Finding the correct foundation is crucial for an all day glow. You want a foundation that will give your client all day coverage, is sweat proof and one that and is suited for her skin type. The right foundation will match the skin tone perfectly. Use a strip test to match her skin to your foundation.

1. Apply foundation with a stiff foundation brush all over the face and down the neck
2. Blend evenly with a light hand to give it an airbrush and luminous finish.

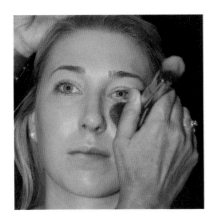

Step 4: Set the Face

Setting your concealer and foundation is an important step in achieving a long lasting makeup application.

1. Use a yellow toned powder to give you a shine free look this will ensure that when your clients wedding photos arrive her face will have the exact same tone as her neck and body.
2. Apply a light dusting to the face, forehead, chin, neck and even the chest if she is wearing a strapless gown.

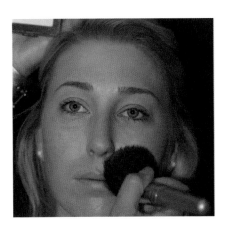

Step 5: Define the Face

Enhance the cheekbones and chin and if she is wearing a strapless dress you will need to tie in her neck to her face.

1. Apply contouring product under the cheekbones with an angled brush for definition.
2. Apply a light dusting below the jaw line to enhance the face.
3. Apply a light layer of bronzer to the neck, chest giving a sun kissed glow.

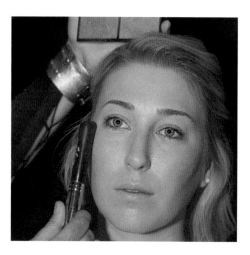

Step 6: A Blushing Bride

For a fresh and luminous bride-to-be glow use the 2-step blush application. Apply a light natural shade of blush to the cheekbones moving in an upward swirl to the hairline followed by a brighter pink or peach shade tapped onto the apples of the cheek, this will brighten your face and give you the blushing bride glow.

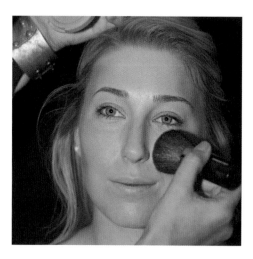

Step 7: Showcase the Eyes

The wedding day is not the time to have heavy smoky eyes or to test out trendy new looks. The wedding day is about an ethereal look that enhances your client's natural beauty. Avoid bright or dark colors, stick to pinks, peaches, light greys or charcoal.

Shadowing

We suggest the following 3-color application

1. Apply a light pink or peach to the floating eyelid.
2. Smoke out the corners of the eye with charcoal grey
3. Highlight the inner corners of the eye and the upper lid just below the brow with a champagne shimmer.

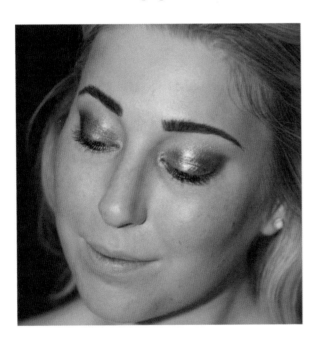

Lining
Try the tight lining technique with your eyeliner to showcase the eyes
1. Line the upper lash line with a dark charcoal or light black
2. 2. Line the lower lash line with the same color
3. Soften the liner by smudging

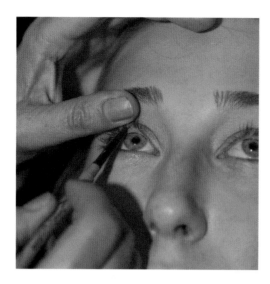

Brows

Defining the eye brows will create a natural frame for the face and make eyes pop in wedding photos. Be sure to use the correct color brow powder or brow pencil to fill-in brows, we suggest a two-color brow process to get a natural look. One colors the same as your clients natural brow color or hair colors the other a lighter color to give the brows definition and depth.

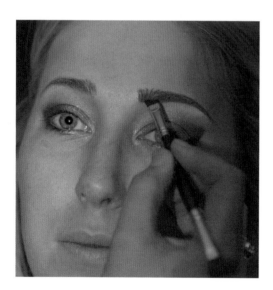

Lashes

Enhancing the lashes will be the final step of your eye makeup application and we recommend suggesting your client get lash extensions if she can afford it or use fiber lash mascara if you can find it. Top off with black waterproof mascara in case there is a spill of a few tears! And if she wants more pop, use the easy technique in the daytime makeup chapter of adding individual lashes to the outer 1/3 corner of the lash line after your mascara application, or you can use the false lash application on your client.

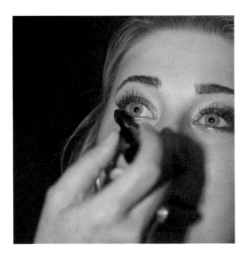

Step 8: Luscious Lips

When it comes to bridal makeup your client's lips matter a great deal. So practice different techniques until you find the look that works well for her and lasts the whole day

1. On her lips, try to use brighter shades of pink, rose or plum colors.
2. Line the lips with a longwearing non-feathering matching shade of lip liner that enhances the color.

We recommend applying a lip stain after you apply the liner and then top it off with lipstick or lip-gloss. Lip stain will ensure that the lip base lasts all day and can be kept up with quick applications of lipstick or lip-gloss.

Have your client use her lipstick throughout the day and keep it handy in an easy to access location and make sure to ask the photographer if the color of lipstick you have chosen will work well with the pictures they are going to take.

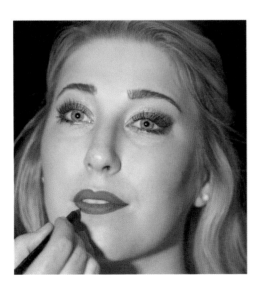

Step 9: Brighten & Highlight

This crucial step creates a glow like no other.

Highlighting the face at the end of your makeup application for a shimmering glamorous glow that will enhance your clients wedding day photos with the illusion of perfect lighting.

1. Use a shimmery powder highlighter below the brow, on the top of the brow bone, and on the top of your cheekbone over the top of your blusher.
2. Apply your powder highlighter to the cupids bow on the top of your upper lip.
3. Then add a small dot of highlighter to the tip of your nose to bring your face forward in pictures.

This is the secret of celebrities who use the camera as their best friend and draw their faces into the sense for beautiful results.

Step 10: Maintain the Glow

Your client needs to know how to keep her look lasting all day and even into the evening. So be sure to council her on how she can maintain her look and keep her glow. You will find this info in the last section of the makeup application chapter.

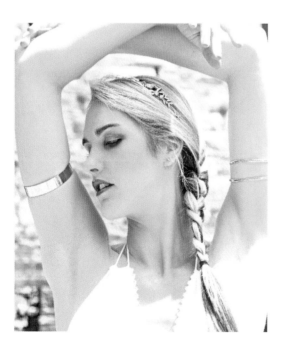

Mature Makeup

As a makeup artist-applying makeup on the mature skin might just be the toughest challenge you will face. That being said it doesn't mean you can't have great success and give your client the gift of glowing beautiful confidence in her appearance. The truth is makeup tends to make us look older so finding the right balance of products that suit her skin and a practiced approach in your makeup application will give her the best results.

How do we help a mature woman look sophisticated and look younger at the same time? The truth is makeup can look good on mature women if you know how to consult with our client and at the same time use the products that enhance their skin and make it look fresh and glowing.

Prep

Before you can even begin your makeup application the client will need to have well-prepared skin and that is in tiptop condition. Exfoliation will improve the skin and it's texture making your makeup application go smoothly. Well-moisturized skin will help to plump up the surface giving you the makeup artist a better canvas to work on. It will be up to you the makeup artist to talk with your client prior to her makeup application and make sure she exfoliates at least two days prior to her makeup session and has well-hydrated skin. This means using a day cream as well as a good night cream along with a serum. She will want to be well hydrated before her makeup application with her recommended daily allowance of water. Water is her skins best friend.

Less is More

This is never truer than when working with mature skin. Less makeup really is the best approach while at the same time so is using the right products for mature skin.

Makeup

Prime: Using a face and eye primer is essential to a makeup application helping to minimize fine lines and pores as well as evening out skin tone and giving you the perfect base to lay down the makeup products. Try to use a silicone-based primer if at all possible; this will give your client the best coverage and foundation for the makeup you apply.

Correct: As with other makeup applications you will have small issues to contend with on the face and it will be no different with mature skin. Often time's mature skin has hyper-pigmentation or age spots, as well as under eye darkness for both of these issues use a lightweight yellow toned corrector and dab it gently over the area working into the skin with your blender or brush. Let the corrector set for a few minutes before applying your foundation. Broken capillaries are another issue with mature skin and must be dealt with before you apply your foundation. The best approach to this issue is to use a green-based corrector and gently dab the corrector into the skin with your blender or a brush. In both cases keep the amount of your corrector to a minimum and always give it time to settle in before applying your foundation.

Foundation: When we work with mature skin it is best to use a liquid foundation that is lightweight and reflective giving your client a dewy look. Heavy cream foundations or powder foundations will only enhance fine lines and wrinkles aging the skin and giving the appearance of covering the face instead of enhancing her beautiful features. Use your foundation brush or beauty blender and gently buff the foundation on to the skin or dab it into the skin with a beauty blender. Never pull the skin with your brush or fingers you will only help to enhance fine lines with this technique.

Concealer: As with the foundation you want the under eye concealer to be liquid and not cream, be sure to use a concealer one shade lighter than your client's skin tone to brighten under the eyes and invoke youthfulness. Use your foundation brush or beauty blender and gently buff the foundation on to the skin or dab it into the skin with a beauty blender.

Powder: Using a setting powder of foundation powder on your mature client is not recommended. It will only enhance fine lines and pores and dull the skin making it look aged and flat.

Blush: Blush is the mature clients best friend, it will give a youthful glow promoting a healthy appearance. You can gently apply a light pink or peach blush to the apples of the cheeks then sweep it back to the temples. Once again use a light hand and layer the product to achieve the blush look you want to create. Do use a powder blush preferably with a little shimmer to it.

Eyes

As with your other makeup applications, the eyes will be the most challenging, the skin on mature eyes is very thin and often has a crêpe like texture. You may even find that mature eyes have become hooded and the floating lid invisible when the eyes are open. To overcome these issues you will want to make sure you have primed the eyes and avoid using heavy or dark shadow colors.

Eye Shadow: Find long wearing shadows that are low in talc content will prevent creasing on the eyelids. I recommend sticking with one color eye shadow in pink, peach, violet or champagne and applying it to the floating lid and coming just above the crease line. Make sure you layer your shadow and blend it out so you don't have a harsh line of demarcation.

Eye Liner: Mature eyes are not always suitable for eyeliners but if your client is used to wearing liner make sure you stay away from a black liner and use a brown or charcoal. I suggest a gel liner that you apply only to the top lash line or tight line on the top lash into the lashes, this will give your clients eye depth and dimension and will be visible if they have hooded eyes.

Mascara: Mascara is essential for ma mature client and I suggest a dark brown shade that is not too harsh. Apply two to three coats lengthening the lashes and focus on the outer corners to give the appearance of larger eyes. Hooded eyes can appear small in size on mature clients and it is up to you to open up the face and bring attention to the eyes.

Brows: More often than not mature women have started to go gray in the brows and you will need to give their brows a boost with a brow product that looks natural and subtle. I suggest using a cream brow product in taupe that you apply with a slanted brow brush and smudge it in with a spoolie. Less is more when it comes to brows but it is still important to do them to give symmetry to the face.

Lips

Mature lips have thin skin and fine lines running out to the face. This happens when our skin starts to lose its collagen and wrinkles start to appear. To overcome this issue you will want to be very attentive to the lips and give them the love they need.

Lip Liner: Mature lips need a lip liner to stop the feathering of lipstick and lip-gloss so make sure you line the lips as well as use a concealer pencil around the edges of the lips to keep the product where it belongs. Apply the concealer from the bow of the lip all the way around the outside then blend into the skin. Apply the lip liner all the way around the lips.

Lipstick: Keep your lipstick subtle and light in color; dark lipsticks tend to make your client's lips look smaller and her face look older. Try pinks or peach based lipsticks and if she is used to dark colors choose a dark mauve to appease her. Top off the lips with a clear gloss or shimmer to give them a youthful glow. Using a lip brush will make the application smooth and crisp.

It will be up to you to educate your mature skin clients on how to apply their products, take care of their aging skin and to stay as hydrated as possible to keep the skin plump and dewy. I always keep a stack of cards for a local esthetician handy to share with my client's who want to seek professional advice from a professional.

Your Set Bag/Makeup Kit

Building your kit should be on the top of your list for building your business and finding the perfect train case to carry it all in is also a critical element. Your case should be easy to haul with enough room and pockets for all of your products. It should be easy to set up when you arrive at your location and give you an element of sophistication.

You are trying to make our first impression a lasting one.

Recommended set bag/makeup kit checklist.

- Quality Brush Set (Powder Brush, Foundation Brush, Blush Brush, Eye Shadow Crease Blending Brush, Flat Eye Shadow Brush, Liner Brush, Lip Brush)
- Brush Cleaner
- A minimum of 4 Liquid Foundations (of the same brand so you can mix easily to get the perfect shade)
- Translucent Setting Powder
- Minimum of 20 Eye shadows (palette form will save you space but loose pigments will give you intense color)
- 3 Blush Colors (peach, pink, plum)
- Lipsticks/Gloss (trendy and popular colors, 2 nudes, 2 pinks, 2 reds, 2 deep colors)
- Lip Pencils (1 nude, 1 pink, 1 red, 1 dark tone)
- 2 Mascaras (1 lengthening mascara, 1 waterproof mascara)
- Eyeliners (black/brown/light brown/white)
- Contour Kit Palette
- Concealer Palette
- False Lashes (assorted lengths and sizes)
- Skin Care Products (moisturizer, makeup remover wipes)
- Primer (face & eye)
- Tools - Eyelash Curler, Lash Glue, Sponges, Q-tips, Spatulas, Tester Wands, Plastic Mixing Palette, Tweezers, Small Scissors, Makeup Brush Belt
- Paper Towels
- Hand Sanitizer
- Client Release Form (hold harmless statement)
- Client Photo Release Form (for portfolio photographs)
- Business Cards
- Tall Folding Chair (if traveling to client)

These are the basic essentials to have in your kit and remember it's better to buy quality than quantity. Being a new business owner it can be hard to get the quality you want at a good price so watch for specials and pay attention to what is happening in the market, it will give you clues to get the best products at the best prices. You can also research companies that let you build your kit at cost effective prices. There are many avenues you can pursue to get your kit filled with the products you want and love.

Try becoming an affiliate for your favorite products or become a distributor for a direct sales line of cosmetics that can give you a second avenue of income in the form of commissions. You are not being a smart businessperson if you are not earning a commission from some of the products you use. You should always be making product recommendations for your clients, I can guarantee they will be asking your opinion on what they should be using. But if you plan to have a great business you need to be able to market and sell a few products that you love and use in your pro kit.

Remember your kit is a reflection of you and is the soul of your business, as such it requires you to pack it in a fashion that is efficient, effective and gives you the creative energy you need to be the best in your business.

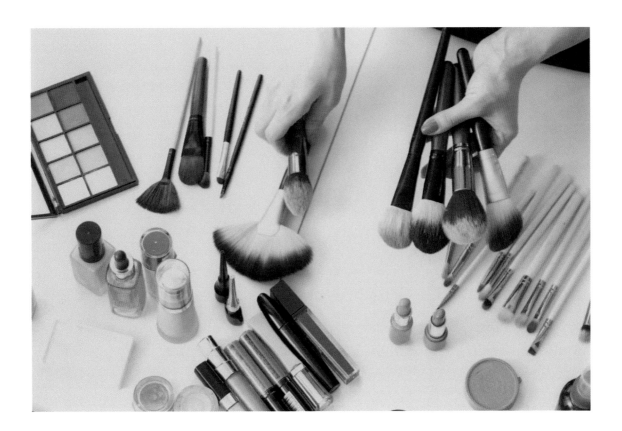

Photography Makeup/HD

Four key elements are necessary to achieve beautiful looking skin in portrait photography: a healthy and rested subject, superior makeup application, good lighting and talented re-touching. Other than recommending a good night's sleep and drinking plenty of water, there's little a photographer can do to change the given subject. A master makeup artist however, can balance skin tones, correct most skin imperfections and even change the perceived shape of a subject's face. Makeup applied well will also boost the effects of good lighting and minimize the work needed later in retouching. Fashion and glamour photographers know the benefits of makeup and usually have a makeup artist on set.

The Tools
Cheap products usually give shoddy results. You don't need to purchase the very best but I do recommend you shop in a reputable makeup store, at the cosmetics counter of a department store, or in a pharmacy with an expanded cosmetics section. Some ideal products can also be purchased online

Brushes and Applicators
I recommend beginning with a kit of three brushes: a face brush, a blush or powder brush, and a concealer or lip brush. A number of companies now make animal-free brushes from bamboo. They are soft, durable, inexpensive, and clean up easily. If you're looking for brushes that can withstand some abuse, spend a little bit more money and purchase good quality synthetic brushes. Be sure, however, that the larger synthetic brushes are very soft and pliable.

Face brush: the largest and fluffiest of makeup brushes, often about 2 inches wide with the bristles curved in a rounded shape

Blush or powder brush: a medium sized, soft brush, 1 to 1.5 inches wide with curved edges. This brush will serve double duty, so avoid purchasing a small blush brush.

Concealer or lip brush: a small brush, about 0.25 to 0.5 inches wide, with ends tapered to a rounded point

Wedge-shaped disposable sponges are handy for all sorts of things. Look for those packaged in a round or square shape, scored to be torn apart into wedges. Beauty blenders are also a great tool to use for applying and blending makeup.

Cotton swabs are indispensable and useful for many tasks. Splurge for a brand-name product with tightly wound swabs. Budget swabs often cause more of a mess than they clean.

Popsicle sticks or tongue depressors are also useful for a number of things. Check your local craft shop for inexpensive boxes of sticks. This is one product to purchase as cheaply as you can.

Disposable hand towels are another indispensable product because tissues are not strong enough. Paper towels are a good second choice but they are not as easy to pack in a small kit.

Blotting film or facial blotting paper is the last disposable item to add to your kit. The films or papers will come in small cardboard packages of about 30 sheets. They are inexpensive and you'll use them a great deal, even if you don't apply any makeup at all.

Cosmetics

You will be able to apply basic makeup with a surprisingly small kit of makeup. You may wish to add more or different products if you find you're often applying makeup, but begin with just the basics.

Translucent loose setting powder: This powder will have a very light skin tone color in the jar but applies neutrally on almost all skin tones. Mineral-based powder is popular and works well. If you are feeling adventurous, mineral-based loose powders can also be purchased with more color. With practice, you can match almost any skin tone by blending from a combination of three, perhaps four, basic shades.

Concealer: This is an inexpensive staple for any makeup kit. You can purchase a small pot of each of three shades of concealer cream (light, medium, and dark), but if you have the patience for shopping, I recommend looking for what is often called a "concealer wheel" or "concealer palette." This single container will contain light, medium, and dark skin tones plus yellow, green, and light purple or pink.

Blush or bronzer: It can be tough picking just one blush or one bronzer that will work on most skin tones, but some companies make both. Blending the two shades will work on skin tones that don't take either the blush or bronzer on their own.

Rice powder: This is a very fine, light, loose white or very pale powder used for absorbing excess oils and highlighting features. Be sure to purchase the real thing and not a chemical substitute. Real rice powder will go on almost invisibly; chemical substitutes will add or change color. If you're unable to find rice powder in the cosmetics shops, try a theatre supply store. This is not an expensive product.

Lip gloss or cream: as with blush and bronzer, it can be difficult to find just one lip color that will look attractive on all skin tones. It's rare that a woman will arrive for a photograph without her lipstick in her purse, and most men would rather give lip treatments a pass. Still, I recommend keeping a pot, squeezable tube, or stick of clear lip-gloss and if you wish, a few tinted lip balms. Do not purchase lip glossin a long container with a stick applicator. It is almost impossible to use gloss this way without contaminating it.

Correcting or Balancing Foundation

With excess oil removed and any blemishes covered, check your client's foundation. Some women are generous in applying foundation or fail to adequately blend foundation along the jaw line. If this is the case with your client, dampen one of your wedge sponges and use it in light gentle strokes to even out the foundation. Pay particular attention to her jawline and hairline, ensuring any makeup lines are smoothly blended out.

When you are ready to apply blush and contour to your client, ask her to smile broadly. Use your medium-sized brush (blush or powder brush) to apply blush from the apex of the apple of her cheeks in a very slight curve down and then up, almost to her ears. Brush the blush on in light strokes, brushing on more makeup in layers until you've achieved a look that is slightly more dramatic than natural.

Next, ask your client to suck in her cheeks. Use your blush or powder brush with your bronzer to lightly apply a bit of contour in the sunken area of her cheeks from about mid-cheek back to hairline. A little contouring goes a long way. When you begin feeling more confident applying contour, consider applying it down the middle of a woman's nose, at her temples, and on the tip of her chin. This will make your client's face look a bit thinner.

Blending

For good makeup application, blend, blend, and blend some more. Begin with your large face brush and lightly sweep in circles to begin to blend in the edges of the blush and contour you've applied. Finish blending by using your face brush to lightly brush on some light flesh colored translucent powder.

Highlight and Manage Shine

Rice powder can be used at this stage both to add some highlights to your client's face and to tone down any shiny areas. To add highlights, use a clean blush or face brush (be sure you've cleaned it of blush and contour), dip the tip of the brush in some rice powder and gently touch the rice powder onto the areas you wish to highlight. Then use your face brush to blend.

Adding highlights to either side of the bridge of your client's nose — near the inside corners of her eyes — will brighten her eyes. To lift a tired look, add a bit of highlighting to the very top of her cheekbones near the bottom of her eye sockets, particularly toward the outer corners of her eyes toward her temples.

If your client has some shiny areas — and this may be all you need to correct for some clients — apply some rice powder on the shine using your face brush. Go lightly; it's easy to over-correct and end up with overly pale looking skin.

Lips

Finish by ensuring your client's lips are smooth, polished, and moist looking. If your client has brought her own lipstick, have her use that. If, however, she did not bring it or her lips need a bit of moisture or shine, use a popsicle stick (or tongue depressor) to scoop a bit of lip gloss out of a pot or to scrape a bit of tinted lip balm off the tube. Apply the gloss or balm from the stick with a clean concealer or lip brush. Don't use your fingers or let your client use her fingers; more gloss or balm will remain on your fingers than on your client's lips.

Applying Makeup to Men

Typically you will limit the makeup application for men to concealing and managing shine, focusing only on problem areas and keeping the make matte and oil free.

Blot and Conceal

Always use blotting paper on a man's skin before applying any concealer. Men naturally produce heavier oil on their faces. If the oil is not blotted, concealer will easily slip off with every attempt to apply it. Otherwise, the same principles for applying concealer to women apply to men. You may only need to be a bit more diligent in blending concealer over shaved facial hair.

Managing Shine

Rice powder works wonderfully to matte shine on a man's face, especially on high foreheads and bald spots. Even if you are not able to completely matte shine in those areas, rice powder will bring the shine down enough that you will have texture to work with in those areas of the photograph when retouching. As with women, apply rice powder to men lightly with a large face brush, blend well, and check to be sure you have not created pasty-white areas.

If your client's skin tone is dark and you are trying to matte significant shine, blend a little tinted translucent powder with the rice powder before applying.

Lips

Some men, particularly those who spend a great deal of time outdoors, have dry or flaking lips. Ask if you might apply a little clear lip balm in this case, or offer it to your client to apply with his finger. This is a circumstance when applying lip balm does work better with a finger. Rub the balm in well; you typically don't want shiny traces on a man's lips.

Clean

Before finishing up, take a close look at your client; remove smudges, makeup flakes, or lint with a cotton swab. Use your face brush or a damp disposable sponge to blend any makeup that needs just a tiny bit more blending

Clean your brushes and cosmetics after every use. Use a conditioning brush spray or isopropyl alcohol on your brushes and cosmetic sanitizer on your cosmetics. Throw away any disposable items you used, and always wash your hands with soap and running water as soon as you are finished.

Stage & Fantasy Makeup

The basic concepts of stage makeup and regular makeup are the same—they are used to create an illusion. Granted, the illusions one wants to create for the stage are typically quite different than those for everyday life. Most often, everyday makeup is simply used to hide blemishes or flaws and highlight one's natural beauty. Stage makeup can be used for dramatic effects and tends to be much heavier than everyday makeup. Today's performer would consider makeup as central to the development of their character as their wardrobe. With the right makeup and skilled application, an actor can become someone entirely different on stage.

What are the Main Differences Between Stage Makeup and Regular Makeup?

The differences between the two aren't as vast as one might think. Stage makeup is meant to be heavier, both in texture and pigment. This allows the makeup effects to be seen from afar, which is typically the case during a stage production. From highlighting and even exaggerating the shape of an actor's face to giving the performer the effects of aging, makeup can transform stage actors.
Regular makeup is much lighter than that which was created for the stage. The pigments are natural looking, giving regular makeup a much more organic look. The idea of regular makeup is to cover blemishes without making the makeup the focal point. Stage makeup should be noticed and is intended to be part of the costume on stage; while everyday makeup is intended more for the background and should blend in to one's natural features.

Can Stage Makeup Be For Everyday Use?

Because stage makeup is essentially just a heavier version of regular makeup, it can be used every day. It's all a matter of personal preference; some people prefer to wear lighter makeup and would most likely be uncomfortable in stage makeup outside of the theater. Wearing it offstage will create a heavier look that is atypical for day-to-day use, but it really is a matter of personal preference.
On the flipside of the debate is this question: can regular makeup be worn on stage? With the right application techniques, regular makeup can work well on stage. By applying the makeup much more heavily and in a more dramatic way, it can create the desired effects just as well as stage makeup. There are also many scenes that require a natural look, making regular makeup a much better choice. It's probably easier to use regular makeup on stage than vice versa. On and off stage, makeup is important in achieving the desired effects and enhancing one's own features. With many different types of makeup to choose from, cream and powder cosmetics play an important role in every stage production as well as in everyday life.
Stage makeup is not limited to face painting only. Rather, stage artists have to apply different types of makeup products for depicting right look as per their character. There are many types of stage makeup that are applied as per the need of show or

event.

For example, in drama, style of makeup is such that characters get appearance like everyday people. On the other hand, in fanciful musical shows, makeup is done for elaborating face and prosthetics like ears. Irrespective of the type of stage makeup, artists have to carry certain tools so that perfect face is created for the show.

Different Types Of Stage Makeup

There are basically two types of stage makeup that are done. These are cream based makeup and cake makeup. Applying cosmetic products that contain oil does cream based makeup. These products come either in cream formula or in stick formats. Cream based makeup is also known as greasepaint. As compared to cake makeup, cream makeup is easier to apply.

Since it is also a heavy makeup, people with sensitive skin can develop acne after four hours of wearing it. Another drawback associated with this type of makeup is that it is harder to remove as compared to cake makeup, which mostly comes in powder form. This powder is mixed with water so as to form a paste for application on face and other body parts.

Cake makeup is gentler on skin. However, applying this type of makeup requires expertise. Both of these types of stage makeup must have high-pigment content, as actors normally perform under bright lights on stage, which reveals imperfections easily. High-pigment makeup helps in concealing blemishes and other skin imperfections.

Apart from other, there are some other types of stage makeup too that are applied. For example, sweat and tears is one of them. This type of makeup is a liquid product that is applied for helping actors in crying and sweating, as per the requirement of show. Similarly, Fake Blood is another style of stage makeup. Actors that appear in supernatural and horror performances mostly use this type of makeup.

Fake blood is used in this makeup for mimicking injuries or some other similar medical conditions. Other types of stage makeup that are also applied to artists are Rainbow Grease Pain, Body Paint and White Face Pain. In rainbow grease pain, grease pain in rainbow colors is applied on the face of artist for drawing exaggerated contours. This type of makeup is also used for painting colorful designs.

Body paint is applied all over the body of artist for making different types of patterns and designs. It is also used for changing the skin tone of artist.While applying makeup to artists, glitters are also used. Glitter may be restricted to face or applied all over the body, it is mostly used by exotic dancers for picking up lights and for producing a sparking effect.

Stage makeup may require years as an assistant or intern. Learning these artistic techniques are time consuming and intensive. If you have a love for art and the ability to stand on your feet for long hours stage makeup might just be the right career path for you.

Face Charts

Unless you are a trained makeup artist chances are you may not know what makeup face charts are or how to use them. Makeup artists use makeup face charts to test out or plan a look for a client, so when meeting with any client use a makeup face chart. They are also used to record a look that has been tried on someone else, like for a photo shoot or bridal trial run. Makeup face charts are very useful to have because they help you keep track of all the different products and color combinations that were used in the application process, in the event that you wish to recreate the look again in the future.

Makeup face charts come on a special type of paper that you can apply makeup directly to, so you want to treat the test face on the paper as an actual person, going through all the steps of applying primer and so forth. Now you can let your creativity soar and experiment by playing around with bronzer, blush, eye colors and lip colors. Spray over the entire look with hairspray once you are finished in order to preserve the look.

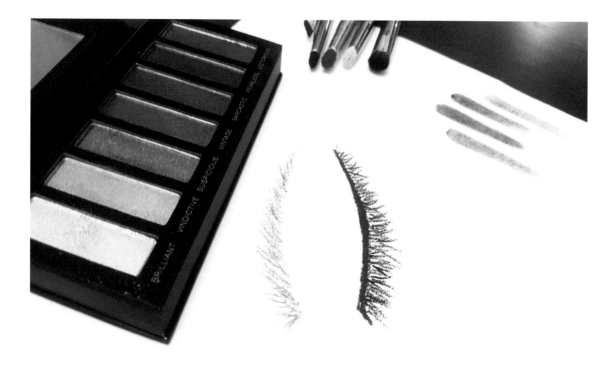

Make-up Chart

Client's name: _____

Foundation: _____
Concealer: _____
Powder: _____
Blush: _____
Bronzer: _____
Contour: _____
Highlighter: _____
Eyeshadows: _____

Eyeliner: _____
Mascara: _____
False Lashes: _____
Brow: _____
Lipliner: _____
Lipstick: _____
Lipgloss: _____
NOTE: _____

Building Your Portfolio

Okay, so you're working on building your portfolio as a makeup artist. Does it include a styled shoot? Should it? What is a styled shoot, anyway? And how do you take part in one?

The Basics

A styled shoot is a specific shoot and it typically involves props, outfits, specific makeup looks, and other details that are arranged around a certain theme. Some shoots are sophisticated, some are retro but often it will be up to the photographer or the team to decide what look they are going for and the mood they are trying to capture. A basic style shoot will require a hair stylist, a makeup artist a photographer a model and the right equipment and location to capture the right look.

Your Portfolio

If you don't have a portfolio of photos then a styled shoot is a great way do trade work for photos building up your portfolio as you build relationships with photographers and models. If you have a large portfolio then a styled shoot is a great way to earn good money. I like styled shoots because it challenges me and lets me be creative, it also allows me to be prepared for the session and come with only the makeup I need to create the look required for the session. Making money is the icing on the cake; styled shoots are fun and exciting. The final outcome of your work will shine when a professional photographer captures your work and spreads the word about your skills as a makeup artist.

Organize a Shoot

If you have gaps in your portfolio then it's time to reach out to some pro photographers and models and start getting a shoot together. This is especially easy if you are great at organizing events and have the ability to work well with others. It will be up to you to plan, organize and execute the shoot but in the end it will be worth the effort.

Who to Invite

- A photographer
- A Model
- Wardrobe stylist
- Hair stylist

A good way to organize a shoot is to start by creating an online style board. A style board will have a series of photos with the theme or idea you want to capture and it will get everyone involved on the same page.

The Event

On the day of the stylized shoot make sure you are well prepared and have every element in place for the outcome you want to achieve. Show up early, be professional and stay until the last person has finished with all of their requirements. You planned it so you are now required to see in through all the way to the end. Once the event is over thank everyone for their time and have the photographer confirm to everyone when the photos will be finished and where they can find them.

No matter what type of shoot you choose keep it short and specific and make sure everyone involved is getting credit for his or her contributions to the shoot. It's not just about you the makeup artist, it is about everyone building a portfolio and creating lasting relationships.

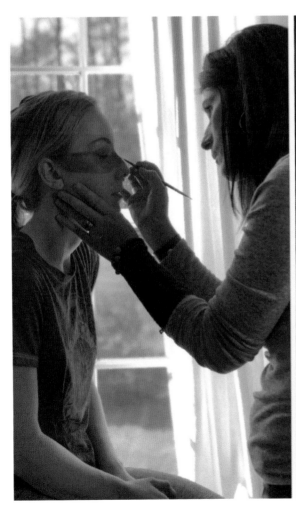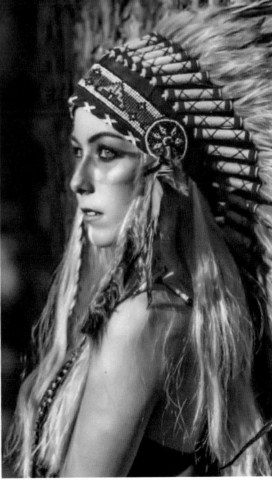

Your New Career

As you embark on your new career in Makeup Artistry and The Business of Makeup Artistry you will be expected to ebb and flow with the whims of those you serve. Preparing yourself to be ready for just about anything in your newly chosen career is very important and at the same time enjoying the journey of this creative career is essential. Having a good attitude and a flexible schedule are just two elements you will need to implement into your new professional life as a makeup artist.

Once you have completed your Master Makeup Artistry course and have gained the skills and knowledge on how to apply makeup, you will need to get a deep understanding of how to own and operate your new makeup business. We recommend buying a copy of *The Business of Makeup Artistry* to help guide you properly into your new career. This guidebook can be found on Amazon and online at the School of Makeup Artistry, we consider it a key element to your success.

The employment opportunities for makeup artists are endless and you are about to set out on a new career full of opportunity, excitement and high income potential.

The future is in your hands and you have the power to design the life of your dreams.

For more info on building your makeup career you can check out *The Business of Makeup Artistry* in paperback or e-book available for download.

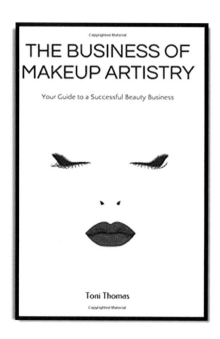

Notes

Printed in Great Britain
by Amazon